"If you are looking for a very practical, user friendly, fact based guide to weight control, this is the book for you."
—Jennifer Miyagawa, Registered Dietitian, *Jenmi Jenmi*

"A slim volume that has the basics of behavior change, and includes all the ones people really struggle with."
—Madelyn Fernstrom, PhD,
Diet and Nutrition Editor for NBC's *TODAY* show

"Every now and then I actually find [a book] I am wildly enthusiastic about. This is one."
—Genene Coté,
nutrition consultant, *Down to Earth Fare*

"Dr. Spencer's book presents a common sense, safe, and enduring weight loss program that presents the essential elements of a healthy lifestyle."
—James E. Gangwisch, PhD,
College of Physicians and Surgeons, Columbia University

"In order to make a permanent change in the obesity statistics in the United States, every dieter must read this book."
—Cascia Talbert, *The Healthy Moms Magazine*

"Stan Spencer gives an excellent account of why people so often overeat. Even more helpful are his many tips on ways to eat smarter and live better."
—Kent Berridge, PhD,
Professor of Psychology, University of Michigan

"An absolute must for anyone who wants to learn how to lose weight permanently. It is the first fat loss book I have read that I cannot fault or disagree with."

—LIAM SARTORIUS, FITNESS AND WEIGHT LOSS COACH

"This book is information-packed! There are hundreds of books written on these topics, but this one brings it all together in one place in a logical format. I will recommend it to my patients."

—DARRIN BANG, DOCTOR OF CHIROPRACTIC

"An excellent book that is well written and evidence based. It will help dispel a lot of the myths that surround weight management."

—GARY MENDOZA, PhD, REGISTERED NUTRITIONIST

"Very informative, and right on target."

—WAYNE WESTCOTT, PhD,
FITNESS RESEARCH DIRECTOR, QUINCY COLLEGE

The Diet Dropout's Guide to

Natural
Weight Loss

The Diet Dropout's Guide to

Natural
Weight Loss

Find Your Easiest
Path to Naturally Thin

Stan Spencer, PhD

FINE LIFE BOOKS

The Diet Dropout's Guide to Natural Weight Loss: Find Your Easiest Path to Naturally Thin

Published by Fine Life Books, Riverside, California
finelifebooks.com

ISBN 978-0-9835717-0-4 (paperback)

Library of Congress Control Number: 2011928360

The *cup* measurement used in the recipes is 240 mL, the *tablespoon* is 15 mL, and the *teaspoon* is 5 mL. A *calorie*, as the term is used in common speech and in this book, is equal to a kilocalorie or Calorie (with a capital C), as those terms are used in scientific research. A Calorie is 4.2 kilojoules.

*To Amy, who is a beautiful testament to the power
of the principles presented in this book.*

Contents

Acknowledgments

I am indebted to many friends, family members, associates, and professionals for their contributions to this book's development.

My sincere thanks to Michelle Bidwell and Marcia Bang for their careful and skillful editing. Thanks to Tina Campbell for bringing the book cover and graphics to life.

I'm grateful to Karen Kuhn, Dale Chadwick, Marilyn Wenzel, Liam Sartorius, Dr. Gary Mendoza, John Jurkiewicz, Chris Smith, Diana Silkwood, Lisa Powell, Julie Rogers, Bill Mercado, Kama Perry, Cindy Clarke, Patricia Lowther, and Betty Kelly Sargent for reading the manuscript and providing helpful comments and encouragement.

Dozens of scientists kindly reviewed those portions of the manuscript referring to their published papers, and several gave additional helpful advice for improving the book. I am especially grateful to Doctors Jack Hollis of Kaiser Permanente, Paul Rozin of the University of Pennsylvania, David Stensel of Loughborough University, J. Wayne Aldridge and Kent Berridge of the University of Michigan, Michael Speca of Alberta Health Services, Ronette Briefel of Mathematica Policy Research, Inc., Graham Horgan of the University of Aberdeen, and Andrew Walley of Imperial College London. Any mistakes or deficiencies that remain are my own.

I thank my mother, Melva Spencer, for her example of healthy cooking with natural ingredients. Thanks to her and my father, George, for supporting and encouraging me in my studies and writing over the years.

Thanks and apologies to my children. The older ones provided helpful comments on the manuscript, and all endured my lack of attention as I spent countless hours researching and writing.

My deepest gratitude goes to my wife, Amy, for tirelessly reviewing and critiquing the manuscript, and for her enduring patience, support, encouragement, and love throughout this project.

Introduction

This is not a diet book. You can lose weight on almost any diet. But diets end, and when they do, the weight returns.

This book is about natural, permanent weight loss. *Natural weight loss* consists of changing the situations, habits, and thought patterns that caused you to gain weight in the first place. If you make those changes *permanent,* your weight loss will be permanent also. That's it. You don't need supplements, specially formulated shakes, surgery, fancy exercise equipment, or any other weight loss product. You don't even need to track calories, follow detailed meal plans, or learn complex recipes. If your ancestors could be thin without following a special diet or buying the latest weight loss product, you can too.

Hundreds of scientific studies relevant to natural weight loss have been conducted over the past few years. This book takes the most useful information from those studies and presents it simply, cutting through diet hype and weight loss myths to provide practical advice for lasting weight loss.

In the short time it will take you to read this book, you will learn thinking and lifestyle habits to help you slim down naturally. With this information, you will be able to create your own weight loss plan—your easiest path to naturally thin—in about five minutes. As you follow the path, you will gradually stop gaining weight and start losing it.

And the best part is, because of the permanent lifestyle changes you are making, the weight won't come back!

Is this book a good match for you? It probably is if:

- you want to get to the root of the problem and address the real reasons for your extra weight, whether they be poor food choices, slow metabolism, emotional eating, out-of-control cravings, or lack of exercise;
- you want to lose weight *permanently,* even if it takes a while; and
- you appreciate books that are brief and to the point.

This book may not be a good match for you if:

- you are looking for a diet or exercise plan; or
- your main goal is to lose weight quickly, even if the weight eventually comes back.

1

Why the Weight?

If this were the early 1960s instead of the 2010s, you might not need a weight loss book. Most people were thin then.

Not now. Even with all the dieting we do, more than two thirds of US adults are now overweight, and the rate of obesity has almost tripled since 1960.[1]

The extra weight isn't natural, nor is it healthy. It not only affects our looks and physical abilities, it increases our risks of developing diabetes, heart disease, stroke, high blood pressure, gallbladder disease, osteoarthritis, sleep apnea, high cholesterol, complications of pregnancy, menstrual irregularities, and cancers of the uterus, breast, colon, and kidney.[1]

So what is behind this weight gain epidemic?

A Less-Active Lifestyle
Our bodies are designed for manual labor and long-distance walking. Many of us, however, enjoy door-to-door motorized transportation to and from a desk job followed by hours of television or other passive

entertainment. Such a lifestyle not only burns few calories but can also encourage us to eat more than we would if we were busy with physical activities.

The Fattening Food Environment

Before processed foods became the norm, our ancestors filled their dinner plates with minimally processed vegetables, fruits, and whole grains. Meats were unprocessed and lean. These natural foods, combined with an active lifestyle, promoted a slim, healthy body.

In contrast to the healthy foods enjoyed by our ancestors, the foods on our grocery store shelves today are often highly processed and have added fat and sugar. These processed foods are packed with calories and are so convenient and tempting that it's easy to eat too much of them.[2,3] As a result, the average adult today eats more calories than in past decades, with most of the extra calories coming from carbohydrate-rich foods such as sweets, soft drinks, potato products, pizza, bread, pasta, and white rice.[4,5]

The average adult today eats more calories than in past decades.

There are ten important aspects of our food environment that encourage us to eat too much.

Foods that Don't Satisfy

Food processing produces calorie-heavy, low-nutrient, low-fiber foods that digest quickly. These foods leave us with loads of calories, soon-empty stomachs, and cravings for more.

Highly Palatable Foods

Highly palatable is a term used by scientists for foods that taste so good that we are tempted to eat them even when our stomachs are full. Most of these are processed foods high in fat, sugar, or refined flour. Such foods have become more abundant and affordable in recent decades, resulting in greater temptations to overeat. We often eat these foods for comfort or pleasure, not because we are hungry.

Highly palatable foods affect the parts of the brain that are responsible for drug addiction and cravings.[6] The authors of a scientific study of the brain's response to highly palatable foods concluded that "overconsumption of palatable food triggers addiction-like...responses in brain reward circuits and drives the development of compulsive eating."[7] In other words, junk food can be addictive.

Calorie-Heavy Foods

While the vegetables, fresh fruits, and whole grains our ancestors ate were high in nutrients and low in calories, the processed foods that fill our grocery store shelves are just the opposite—high in calories and low in nutrients. The result is that a typical meal of modern processed foods has more calories than we need and often too few nutrients. Calorie-heavy foods are believed to be a major factor in the weight gain epidemic.[8]

Cheap, Convenient Food

There is inexpensive, ready-to-eat food almost everywhere we go. We have candy jars at work and cookie jars at home. We stock our refrigerators with soft drinks and our pantries with packaged snacks. Just seeing junk food can make us hungry, and food within easy reach is harder to resist than food that requires a little more effort to obtain.[9,10] Eating too much has never been easier.

Large Portions

In the US, portion sizes of many foods have increased two- to five-fold since the 1970s.[11] We tend to keep eating until the portion in front of us is gone, no matter what its size. Similarly, we tend to eat more when eating a snack food directly out of a large package (such as a bag of potato chips) than when served individual portions.[10]

Passive Entertainment

Watching television or movies burns very few calories. It also encourages needless eating. If we eat during such entertainment, our distraction with the storyline can cause us to continue eating past the point at which we would normally be satisfied.[10]

Convenient Substitutes for Water

Sports drinks, sugary soft drinks, fruit juices, and alcoholic drinks are readily available in our homes and elsewhere. These drinks quickly add calories without lasting satisfaction. Their consumption is believed to be a major factor in the weight gain epidemic.[2,12]

Misleading Labels and Advertising

A picture of a slender athlete on a package of fresh fruit might make sense. The same picture on an "energy bar" consisting mostly of corn syrup and puffed rice does not. Advertisements often inaccurately depict the health benefits of the foods they are promoting.

Unhealthy Snack Foods

Common snack foods tend to be higher in calories and lower in nutrients than the kinds of foods usually eaten with meals.[12] They are quick to add calories but slow to satisfy.

Restaurants

We eat out more now than in decades past.[12] Restaurant food tends to be higher in calories and served in larger portions than food cooked at home. As a result, one restaurant meal might have enough calories for an entire day.

The Solution

Think of excess fat as a collection of bad habits. Lose the fat-promoting habits, and you will lose the excess fat. Each time you give up one of these bad habits (all other things being equal), you will lose fat until your body naturally settles at a lower weight. At that point you will need to give up another bad habit to lose more weight and keep it off.

Think of excess fat as a collection of bad habits.

Permanent weight loss requires permanent lifestyle changes.[13] The information in this book will help you replace bad habits with good ones and make the lifestyle changes required for lasting weight loss. You will learn how small adjustments in your eating and exercise habits can result in a big difference in body fat over time, why many of the things you hear about gaining or losing weight are false, and why popular diets rarely produce permanent weight loss. You will also learn how to change your personal environment so it's no longer fattening, boost your metabolism without drugs or supplements, give your body the exercise it needs without wasting time, eat fewer calories without counting them or going hungry, and beat temptation with the willpower you already have.

Often, the hardest part of forming new habits is just getting started. Watch for the **QuickStart Tips** as you read through the book. They will prompt you to pause and take solid steps down the path to your naturally thin potential.

2
Why Diets Fail

Besides emptying your pocketbook, the main problem with most popular diets is they give you an excuse to put off making the *permanent* changes in lifestyle and thinking you need for lasting weight loss.[1]

You can lose weight with any diet that restricts calories, and all you have to do to keep the weight off is stay on the diet. In reality, though, most diets are so unpleasant, inconvenient, boring, complex, or expensive that they are difficult to stick with for very long.[2] As you fall back into old habits, you regain the weight. After slipping back to the same old weight two or three times, you start to believe that it must be your "natural" weight, and you quit trying altogether.

Most diets are difficult to stick with for very long.

A group of University of California researchers reviewed scientific studies of the long-term effects of dieting. They found that most of the weight dieters lost was regained within four or five years. In fact, in some of the studies they analyzed, a history of dieting appeared to lead to *more* weight gain, not less, over time. They concluded that dieters who manage to keep the weight off "are the rare exception rather than the rule" and that "there is little support for the notion that diets lead to lasting weight loss or health benefits."[3]

Top health experts agree that lasting weight loss for most people is best accomplished by making permanent changes in eating habits and physical activity.[4] Changing habits takes time, but without real lifestyle changes, any weight you lose will soon return.

If you are well read in weight loss literature, you may already be familiar with much of the information presented in this book. Whatever your level of prior knowledge, I hope you will find some tools that help you convert your knowledge into healthier habits and a slimmer lifestyle.

3
Emotional Eating
(And How to Quit)

When we eat highly palatable foods (foods high in fat, sugar, or refined flour), our brain's reward circuitry is activated, producing pleasure and desire.[1,2] These effects motivated our ancestors to load up on high-calorie foods in times of plenty in order to endure times of food scarcity. For them, taking advantage of available high-calorie food was a matter of survival. We, on the other hand, don't usually need the extra calories. This reward circuitry motivates us to keep eating anyway, just as it motivates the drug addict to continue his self-destructive behavior.[3,4]

When we are surrounded by highly palatable foods, it's easy to overuse this reward circuitry. We use the natural highs that these foods give us to comfort ourselves when we are stressed, anxious, bored, sad, frustrated, or depressed. We often eat to regulate our emotions, not because we are hungry. This is called *self-medicating* or *emotional eating*. While using food for emotional comfort once in a while is not necessarily a bad thing, making a habit out of it is a recipe for continued weight gain.

Finding better ways to manage your emotions can help you overcome a habit of emotional eating. In this chapter you will learn five ways to improve your emotional well-being: *focusing on the present, mental relaxation, healthy thinking, social interaction,* and *doing something productive.*

Focus on the Present

Harvard psychology researchers did a study with over two thousand iPhone users to find out what kinds of thoughts and activities make people happy. The researchers created an iPhone app to prompt the study participants at random times as they went about their daily lives.[5] Each time they were prompted, the participants reported what they were doing, thinking, and feeling. Participants who had been mentally focused on whatever they were doing or experiencing generally reported feeling happier than those whose minds had been wandering. Even daydreaming about pleasant topics was less often associated with happiness than was focusing on the present task or experience.

Whether you are at your job, doing housework, playing a sport, or taking a walk, focusing your mind on your present activity or experience can help elevate your mood.

As you focus on the present, try to keep an accepting, nonjudgmental attitude toward whatever you are experiencing at the moment. This practice, called *mindfulness*, has been taught in Eastern traditions for centuries, and is increasingly used in Western medicine to treat anxiety, depression, addictions, eating disorders, and stress-related conditions.[6]

You can practice mindfulness now by taking a moment to look around and notice the colors, sounds, and other details of your environment. As you become caught up in the present, you free your mind from the worries and unhealthy thought patterns that depress your mood.

Try to practice mindfulness throughout the day. When you are actively engaged in a task, keep your mind on that task instead of letting your thoughts wander. When you are not actively engaged in a task, focus your thoughts on your present experience or surroundings.

The most difficult part of focusing on the present is just remembering to do it. You can use a card like the sample one at the end of the chapter as a reminder. Place it where you will see it often, and move it around every day or two so it doesn't fade into the background.

Relax Your Mind

When you are in a stressful situation, your body experiences a *stress response* (often called the "fight or flight" response). Your heart rate and blood pressure increase, your air passages open up, and glucose pours into your blood stream. Blood vessels that feed your skin and digestive system constrict, sending extra blood to your muscles, heart, and brain. These changes prepare your body and mind for action. You are on edge, ready to fight or flee.[7]

The stress response is natural and sometimes beneficial. It enables you to focus your physical and mental abilities in a sudden dangerous or challenging situation. The constant activation of the stress response, however, is not natural, and can cause various mental and physical problems.[8]

Your body also has a *relaxation response* that opposes the stress response. The relaxation response occurs naturally when your mind is at ease, but it can't occur when you are worrying, judging, or analyzing. You can deliberately produce the relaxation response by freeing your mind from these kinds of thoughts. One way to do this is by meditating. Sleeping, lounging around, and watching television are often less helpful because they may not free your mind from disturbing or arousing thoughts.

Regular activation of the relaxation response can reduce stress, anxiety, and depression and promote healing from stress-related physical illnesses.[8,9] Daily mental relaxation will increase your ability to tolerate the stressful events in your life as they occur, so you are less tempted to turn to food for comfort.[8]

There are several ways to activate the relaxation response. Three of the easiest and most powerful techniques are *sensory focus, basic meditation,* and *repetitive physical exercise.* These all involve focusing your mind on something simple and non-arousing. This gives your brain an intellectual and emotional break, allowing the relaxation response to occur. Here's how to get started on a more relaxing lifestyle:

1. Read the rest of this section, then choose a mental relaxation technique (sensory focus, basic meditation, or repetitive physical exercise) and make it a daily habit.

2. Choose a set time each day for your relaxation session, such as after your morning shower or during an afternoon break.

3. To allow the relaxation response to fully engage, make your daily relaxation session last for at least twelve minutes.[9] If you don't have time for a twelve-minute session, do at least a five-minute session so you don't get out of the habit.

4. Use one or more of these mental relaxation techniques to calm yourself any time you start to feel stressed or anxious throughout the day.

Sensory Focus

Sensory focus is a way of focusing on the present (as discussed previously) in which you limit your focus to a physical sensation or perception.

You are practicing sensory focus when you are engrossed by the colors of a sunset or carried away by the sounds of ocean waves. The object of your focus, however, doesn't need to be as spectacular as a sunset or ocean waves. Here are some simple ways to do sensory focus:

- Watch the dancing flames of a fireplace or candles.

- Listen to calming instrumental music simply to enjoy it, without analyzing or judging it.

- Enjoy the warmth of a bath.

- Touch with your fingertips the various surfaces within your reach, noticing the texture and temperature of each. Slide your fingers along each surface and notice any changes in form or texture.

As your sensory focus displaces other thoughts, you will begin to relax. Inevitably, however, your mind will wander and thoughts of other matters will intrude, especially in the beginning. Instead of analyzing or trying to suppress these thoughts, simply think, "Oh, well," and return your attention to your sensory focus.[9] Don't worry about how well you are doing. The important thing is to just keep returning your attention to your sensory focus whenever your mind wanders.

Daily mental relaxation will increase your ability to tolerate the stressful events in your life as they occur.

Progressive muscle relaxation is another form of sensory focus. It consists of focusing on the feelings of tension and relaxation in your muscles as you flex and relax different muscle groups. Start by tensing the muscles in your toes and feet for a few seconds. Now let them relax, noticing the release of tension. Do the same with the muscles of your calves, thighs, abdomen, hands, arms, shoulders, neck, and face, tensing and then relaxing each set of muscles in turn.

Basic Meditation

Meditation is sustained mental focus on a thought or sensation. For your meditation to be relaxing, the thought or sensation should be neutral or positive. The relaxation response occurs naturally as your meditation clears your mind of the thoughts and worries that keep you stressed.

Basic meditation is simply a particular way of doing sensory focus: it is usually done by focusing on your breathing while sitting in a quiet place with your eyes closed.

Before you begin a meditation session, it may be helpful to do a minute or two of progressive muscle relaxation. This will help you get physically comfortable and break away from your current train of thought.

When you are comfortable, begin your meditation by directing your attention to your breathing. Notice each breath as it enters and then leaves your body. Don't try to control your rate of breathing. It will become slower on its own as you relax. Whenever your mind wanders, think, "Oh, well," and return your attention to your breathing.

**Meditation is sustained mental focus
on a thought or sensation.**

You can help yourself maintain focus during basic meditation by silently saying a positive or neutral focus word, such as *peace* or *one*, each time you breathe out. A focus word is like a broom that sweeps intruding thoughts from your mind each time you repeat it. Draw the focus word out ("onnnnne") to match the length of the breath.

Continue meditating for at least twelve minutes, then remain seated a little longer to enjoy the relaxation before you gradually transition into your next activity.

Take a moment now and then throughout the day to direct your attention to your breathing and recall the relaxation you experienced during your meditation session.

If you are finding it difficult to focus on your breathing during a meditation session, try focusing on tactile sensations instead. Place a hand on an article of your clothing and slowly move your fingers one at a time in rhythm with your breathing. As you move each finger, notice the texture of the fabric and repeat your focus word.

When first trying basic meditation, most people experience one of three outcomes: mental relaxation, sleepiness, or anxiety.

Mental relaxation is, of course, the desired outcome. Your ability to relax while meditating will improve with practice.

If you have trouble staying awake, try meditating at a different time, and certainly not just before bedtime. Sit up and keep your back straight. You want a position that is comfortable but not one that signals to your brain that you are preparing for sleep. Be patient. It may take struggling through several meditation sessions to get your brain out of the habit of entering sleep mode whenever you slow down and close your eyes.

Anxiety can result from the thoughts that intrude as you try to meditate: thoughts of things you forgot to do, wish you hadn't done, or are afraid might happen. Every time such thoughts arise, simply return your focus to your breathing or other sensory anchor. Tell yourself that this is your time to relax; the distracting thoughts can wait.

Anxiety may also result from worrying about how well your meditation is going. Don't worry. Simply sitting down and going through the motions of meditation is beneficial, however frustrating it may be. Every time you practice you'll get a little better at ignoring the distracting thoughts and staying focused.

Meditation-based therapy has been used successfully in the treatment of chronic pain, stress, anxiety, and depression.[10] The effects of meditation on the brain are real and persist beyond the meditation session. In a 2010 study, researchers used magnetic resonance imaging (MRI) to look at the brains of twenty-six people before and after participation in an eight-week meditation class.[11] Participants practiced meditation for about twenty minutes a day during the eight-week period. At the end of the class, participants reported that their stress levels had decreased substantially, and MRI images showed actual physical changes in an area of their brains associated with stress and anxiety.

Repetitive Physical Exercise

There is growing evidence that exercise is an effective treatment for both depression and anxiety, and that it can provide protection from the harmful consequences of stress.[12,13] The reasons for these benefits aren't entirely clear,[14] but it's likely that they are partly due to the ability of exercise to activate the relaxation response.

Focusing your mind on any simple, repetitive movement or sensation can activate the relaxation response. When you have such a focus during exercise it becomes meditation in motion.

While doing almost any exercise, you can focus your attention on your muscles contracting, your body's movements, or the rhythm of your breathing. To help keep your mind free of distracting thoughts, repeat a focus word or phrase with each repetition or stroke of your exercise.

Work activities such as hoeing weeds, mowing a lawn, or vacuuming a floor can also provide the simple focus needed to activate the relaxation response. Physical activities that require intense concentration or bursts of energy, such as basketball and tennis, are not as effective.[9]

Forms of exercise that emphasize mindfulness, such as yoga, tai chi, and qigong, may be especially helpful. Taking a class in one of these techniques can also give you the benefit of group support.

Think Healthfully

Negative emotions such as sadness, fear, anger, and concern are natural and can serve useful functions by motivating us to take action. Often, however, we experience these emotions needlessly or excessively because of unhealthy thinking habits. When negative emotions are extreme or chronic, they are not helpful and can increase the temptation to self-medicate with food.

Thoughts influence emotions, and irrational thinking can lead to unhealthy emotional states. When something doesn't go your way, it's easy to fall into one of the following irrational thought patterns:

- *Demanding fairness or justice.* "That shouldn't have happened." "It wasn't fair." "Why me?" Life often isn't fair. Things often won't go your way, and people who wrong you will often go unpunished, no matter how much you seek justice. Expecting life to always be fair is not only irrational but also adds disappointment to the injustices you suffer.

- *Catastrophizing.* "It's awful that this happened." When something unfortunate happens, focusing on how bad it is doesn't help your emotional state or your ability to handle the situation. It's better to think of misfortune in shades of gray rather than black or white. It could have been better *or* worse.

- *Hopelessness.* "I can't stand it." "I can't handle this." The truth is that you have been able to stand everything that has happened in your life so far. You are living proof of that.

- *Condemning or blaming.* "I'm so stupid." "What an idiot he is." Condemning or assigning blame doesn't fix anything. No matter who is to blame for an unfortunate situation, you are the one responsible for your emotional reaction to it.

As you free yourself from these irrational thought patterns and practice a more rational, healthy way of thinking, your mental state will improve and you will be less controlled by emotions. There are three attitudes that can help you develop healthy thinking habits: *emotional independence, perspective,* and *acceptance.*

Emotional Independence

Your emotions are not determined by what others think, say, or do. Your anger, chronic anxiety, and depression are not caused by other people or even by your circumstances, but by how you *think* about those people or circumstances. *No one can make you feel any emotion without your consent.*

Don't take the thoughtless behavior of others personally, even if you believe it was meant to be personal. You can take things seriously (i.e., learn from them) without taking them personally (i.e., allowing them to control how you feel about yourself).

Perspective

Put negative situations in perspective and be grateful for what you have. A little change in perspective can make a big emotional difference.

When something "bad" happens to you, how bad is it really? Let's use an analogy of damage to your physical body. What is one of the worst things that could happen to your body? Losing all four limbs? Let's call that 100 percent bad. How about having both hands cut off? Maybe 50 percent bad. A disfiguring facial scar? Maybe 40 percent. Two broken legs and a crushed foot? Maybe 20 percent. A smashed finger? Maybe 2 percent. A stubbed toe? Probably less than 1 percent.

Now use this scale to rate any undesirable situation you find yourself in. What "percent bad" is it? Most undesirable things that happen in the course of a week will probably rate less than 1 percent bad. Compared with real tragedies, 1 percent isn't that bad, is it? You can certainly handle 1 percent bad. When something happens that is not your preference, ask yourself how bad it really is, and be happy that things are not worse.

Another way to quickly gain perspective is to stop and think about the good things in your life. Make a list of ten things you are thankful for and keep it where you can refer to it when you are feeling down. See the sample card at the end of the chapter. Think of how easily you could lose some of those things, and how blessed you are to have them. Choose to see the glass as half full rather than half empty.

Ask yourself if what you are stressing over today will matter a year from now.

Acceptance

There are some things you can't change. The past is one thing that can't be changed, no matter how much you dwell on it. There are other things that could be changed but aren't worth the effort or cost. If you can't or choose not to change something, accept it as it is.

Nobody's perfect. Accept imperfection in yourself, others, and circumstances, even as you work to make positive changes. When you are feeling bad about yourself, repeat, "I accept myself, imperfect though I am, fully and completely." Accept other people in the same way.

Acceptance also means accepting your emotions. It's OK to be sad sometimes, or angry, lonely, frustrated, or hungry. These emotions are part of what it means to be human. We aren't meant to be comfortable and content all of the time. When you feel unpleasant emotions, remind yourself that emotions change, and you will probably feel better soon.

Change Your Way of Thinking in One Day

Your ultimate goal is to control your emotional reaction to a situation by changing the way you look at it. The three-step routine below can help you kick your habit of irrational thinking and become a happier person in a single day.

Choose a day to practice. On that day, every time you find yourself dwelling on an unpleasant situation or having irrational thoughts, stop and take a few minutes to apply each of the three healthy attitudes:

1. *Emotional independence.* Remind yourself that your emotions are caused by your own thoughts and that no one can make you feel any emotion without your consent.

2. *Perspective.* Ask yourself what "percent bad" the situation is. Be grateful for what you have, and that things are not worse.

3. *Acceptance.* Decide what aspects of a negative situation can be realistically changed, and accept the rest as your new reality.

Remind yourself that no one is perfect, and everyone has difficulties. Accept yourself even as you try to do better. Accept others the same way. Accept your emotions as the temporary manifestations that they are.

Going through these three steps every time you have irrational thoughts will be time-consuming and inconvenient. That's OK; do it anyway. You will soon notice yourself stopping irrational thoughts before they are fully formed, just to avoid the bother of going through the routine. You will also quickly improve your healthy thinking skills.

You can kick your habit of irrational thinking and become a happier person in a single day.

Be a Card-Carrying Healthy Thinker

No matter what you do, unpleasant things happen in your life. When they do, choose *not* to think, "That never should have happened; it's awful that it did; I just can't handle this; someone should suffer for it!" Train yourself to instead think, "I wouldn't have chosen it, but it happened, and now it's my new starting point, whether justice is done or not. It's only X percent bad, and I can handle that. I alone determine how this situation will affect me emotionally."

Use a card like the one at the end of the chapter as a reminder to practice healthy thinking. A habit of healthy thinking will help you handle daily challenges and annoyances without needing to turn to food for comfort.

Interact Socially

Humans are naturally social creatures. To be happy, we need to interact with others. Here are some ways to get more social interaction:

- Visit with a family member or friend.

- Join a team or club.

- Help others. Reaching out to serve others can help you keep your mind off your own troubles and lift your spirits.

- Get together with other people who share your interests, or develop some new interests that you can enjoy with others.

- Join a twelve-step recovery program. Being active in a twelve-step group can help you feel connected and understood.

- Get a pet to interact with and care for.

Do Something Productive

The personal fulfillment you feel when you develop a new skill, create something useful or beautiful, or help others can increase your self-esteem, brighten your outlook, and improve your emotional health. Doing something productive can also make you a more interesting person, expanding your opportunities for social interaction. Make an effort to develop new interests and have new experiences. Variety and change are important for keeping yourself refreshed and excited about your activities.

QuickStart Tip—*At fatlossscience.org/book you can find a printable version of the reminder card on the next page. Cut along the outer lines and fold along the inner lines to make a tri-fold, wallet-sized card.*

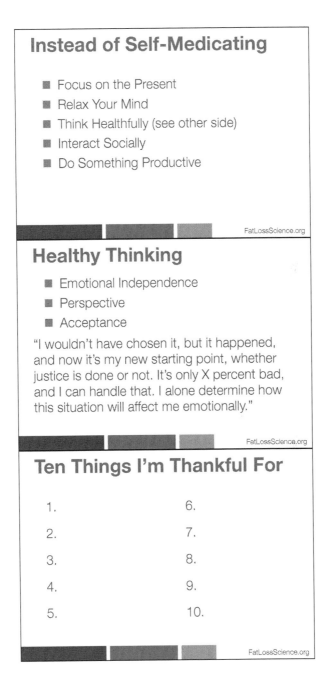

Instead of Self-Medicating

- Focus on the Present
- Relax Your Mind
- Think Healthfully (see other side)
- Interact Socially
- Do Something Productive

FatLossScience.org

Healthy Thinking

- Emotional Independence
- Perspective
- Acceptance

"I wouldn't have chosen it, but it happened, and now it's my new starting point, whether justice is done or not. It's only X percent bad, and I can handle that. I alone determine how this situation will affect me emotionally."

FatLossScience.org

Ten Things I'm Thankful For

1.   6.

2.   7.

3.   8.

4.   9.

5.   10.

FatLossScience.org

4

Beat Temptation
(With Minimal Willpower)

In the previous chapter, you learned how to manage your emotions in order to avoid the need to eat for emotional comfort (emotional eating). In this chapter, you will learn how to avoid eating in response to external temptations, such as the sight or smell of a favorite food, sometimes called *external eating*. Not surprisingly, habitual external eating is associated with excess weight gain.[1]

If you have a habit of external eating, you can overcome it by learning to avoid food temptations and to quickly calm your cravings whenever you are tempted.

Two Keys to Avoiding Temptations

It's usually easier to avoid temptations than to resist them. The best way to avoid food temptations is to clean up your environment. Another way is to decide in advance what you will do in situations that normally tempt you.

Clean Up Your Personal Environment

There are many little things you can do to remove temptations from your environment. Here are a few:

- Keep junk food out of the house as much as possible.

- If you must have junk food in your house, keep it out of sight.

- Remove temptations from your space at work.

- Start a grocery list of healthy food choices. Read chapter 6 and the appendices at the back of the book for ideas.

- Designate an eating area and don't eat anywhere else, then stay out of the eating area as much as possible when it isn't mealtime.

- Avoid places where you will be tempted by unhealthy foods. This may mean changing your route to work, the places you shop, or the aisles you walk down in the grocery store.

- Expose yourself to fewer commercials for unhealthy foods by watching less television.

Decide in Advance

Next time you walk by the candy jar on your coworker's desk, are you going to take a sample? Don't wait until you are in the midst of temptation to decide. Decide now.

Efforts at resisting temptation are often undermined by rationalizing. ("Just one piece of candy won't hurt. I've been good all morning. I deserve a reward.") When you have already made a firm decision and rehearsed your response ahead of time, you can act quickly in a tempting situation, leaving no time for rationalizing.

A temptation is a decision that has not yet been made. Once you have truly decided that eating candy at work isn't an option, the candy jars will fade into the background and won't be so tempting.

Another reason to make food decisions in advance is that the mere sight or smell of highly palatable foods can bring on cravings that reduce your ability to think clearly and make choices you won't regret the next day.

Here are some examples of decisions you may want to make in advance:

- How many servings of sweets will you eat each day?
- What will you do instead of eating when you feel stressed?
- Will you snack while watching television or reading?
- Will you snack at all? If so, when? What will you eat?
- How often will you buy junk food?
- What will you do when offered a piece of candy or other unhealthy snack between meals? Politely decline it? Accept it, but save it to eat with your next meal?

Once you have made these decisions, write them down, and put the list where you will see and notice it. Review your decisions often. Your aim is to make your responses to previously tempting situations automatic.

A temptation is a decision that has not yet been made.

If you don't always follow through with your decisions, don't beat yourself up over it. Nobody is perfect. Just keep up the effort. You haven't failed until you've given up. Every bit of improvement will help you in your weight loss goals.

It can also be helpful to decide what you will eat for each meal a day in advance, and get as much of it ready as you can ahead of time, *before* you get hungry.

Nine Ways to Calm Cravings

One way external temptations lead to overeating is by causing cravings,[2] which can wear down even the strongest resolve. Knowing how to calm cravings quickly can make a big difference in your eating habits. Here are some important facts to remember about food cravings:

- Cravings are normal, especially for those who are dieting or attempting to restrict particular foods.[3] They are nothing to feel guilty or concerned about.

- Having a craving doesn't mean you're hungry. One difference between food cravings and hunger is that food cravings tend to be highly specific, involving intense desires for specific foods, while hunger produces a more general desire to eat almost any food that is available. Chocolate, ice cream, cookies, bread, and salty snacks are commonly craved foods. If only ice cream will do, it's a craving, not hunger.

- Common cravings are generally not indicative of specific nutritional needs, but are better explained by various psychological theories.[3] Your body doesn't need the food you crave. It is only that your brain desires it.

- Cravings don't last forever. You don't need to give in to a craving, and you don't need to completely eliminate it. All you really need to do is outlast it. Outlasting a craving doesn't have to be difficult. You just need the right tools.

If you do an Internet search for "cravings," you will find dozens of suggestions for calming them: take a walk, take a nap, eat some nuts, write in your journal, visit with a friend, exercise. Most of those ideas may work fine if you aren't driving to work through the doughnut district or sitting in a staff meeting in front of a plate of chocolate chip cookies. Here are eight mental tools you can use to calm cravings anywhere, anytime, and a ninth tool (taking a brisk walk) that works very well when you are able to use it.

Focus Your Thoughts on Something Else

A craving is generally prompted by the sight or smell of a favorite food, or by an unpleasant emotion that brings on thoughts of a comfort food. When you continue to think of the craved food, you keep the craving alive. Your thoughts usually involve visual images—if you are craving doughnuts, you probably have an image of a doughnut in your mind. Now here's the key to calming the craving: the part of your mind that holds visual images can hold only one image at a time. If you deliberately imagine something else, the new image will displace the image of the craved food, and your craving will gradually diminish.[4]

Sometimes, however, your craving is so strong you are unable to think about anything else long enough for the craving to subside. In those situations, use a sensory focus technique from chapter 3. Next time you have a food craving, try this. Without looking at your hand, touch an article of your clothing. Find a seam and move your fingers across it. Notice the changes in form and texture that you feel. As you do so, images of the fabric will enter your mind and displace the mental image of the food you are craving. Continue this exercise for about a minute, or until the craving is gone.

Remember What You Really Want

If you don't really want to lose weight, you won't have much success, no matter how much effort you put into it. You will find ways to sabotage your own efforts and keep the weight on.

Perhaps you are afraid of the attention or higher social expectations that having a more attractive body might bring. Maybe you are afraid that if you lose weight, you will no longer fit in with your friends, or that you will be rejected by family members. Maybe the extra weight helps you feel safe. Maybe being thin just doesn't seem to be worth the extra effort that will be required. If you don't really want to have a slimmer body, this book won't do you much good.

On the other hand, if you really *do* want to lose weight, the emotional power of this desire can help you counter your cravings. Spend a few minutes and put your specific weight loss goal, and reasons behind your goal, on paper. Write on a small card what you really want (to be a certain weight or size, for example) and why you want it. Your motives might include health, relationship, or emotional benefits, physical goals (such as a desired hiking vacation), or other reasons. See the sample card at the end of this chapter.

When you experience a craving, look at the card, think about what you really want and why, and ask yourself if giving in to the craving would help you get there. Give it some serious thought for at least a minute, or until the craving is gone.

You can also use this tool to head off cravings before they occur. If you know you are going to be in a situation that prompts cravings, look at your card and spend a minute or so remembering your weight loss goal and reasons, then keep those motivating thoughts in mind as you pass through the tempting situation.

See the Food in a Different Light

Advertisers often use imagery to manipulate your perception of foods and induce cravings. You turn the page of a magazine and see a picture of a chocolate-glazed doughnut bathed in soft light, over a white tablecloth, poised next to a pair of luscious red lips. You can almost taste the glistening icing. You suddenly crave doughnuts.

You can use your own mental imagery to see the doughnut in a different, less flattering light, so it no longer seems so desirable. Try this. In your imagination, replace the red lips with a pair of doughnut-devouring maggots. (I'm making this up, and so can you.) Imagine a spot of green mold on the side of the doughnut. Replace the white tablecloth with a dirty sidewalk, the doughnut surrounded by flattened, blackened pieces of discarded chewing gum. Now imagine taking a bite of it. Taste the bitter mold. Keep this up for about a minute, or until the craving is gone.

Imagine Eating More than You Want

Carnegie Mellon University researchers conducted a pair of experiments that demonstrated how your imagination can affect your cravings.[5] In one experiment, they instructed a group of participants to imagine moving three M&M's candies, one at a time, from one bowl to another. A second group of participants was instructed to imagine moving thirty M&M's. After completing their assigned visualizations, all of the participants were allowed to eat as much as they wanted from a bowl of real M&M's. As you might expect, the participants who had imagined moving thirty M&M's ate more real M&M's, on average, than those who had imagined moving only three. After all, they had spent more time thinking about the candies and were probably experiencing stronger cravings.

In the other experiment, researchers instructed one group of participants to imagine *eating* three M&M's, one at a time, and a second group to imagine eating thirty. The participants were then allowed to eat as many real M&M's as they wanted. This time the results were different: the participants who had imagined eating thirty M&M's ate *fewer* real M&M's than those who had imagined eating only three.

This study showed that, while simply thinking about junk food can increase your desire for it, thinking about eating *enough* of the food can have the opposite effect, so that you end up eating less.

Are you still craving that chocolate-glazed doughnut from the previous section? If so, imagine eating one: take a bite, chew it, smell it, taste it, swallow it, and feel it sitting heavily in your stomach. Now take another bite. When you are finished with that doughnut, imagine eating another one, and another. Keep this up until you are thoroughly bored with the exercise. Has your craving diminished?

If you want to speed things along, combine this tool with the previous one. At the end of every imagined mouthful, visualize a bit of mold and imagine tasting something bitter. You will get your fill of doughnuts sooner.

Count the Exercise Cost

A 20-ounce (591-mL) bottle of sugary soda contains about 250 calories, which would take nearly a half hour of jogging or an hour of brisk walking to burn off (for a 150-lb or 70-kg adult). The 40 calories in *one* medium-sized bite of chocolate would take about ten minutes of brisk walking to erase.

In a 2012 study, researchers created a sign with the words "Did you know that working off a bottle of soda or fruit juice takes about 50 minutes of running" and posted it in a corner store frequented by thirsty adolescents. The presence of the sign reduced the odds that an adolescent would purchase a sugar-sweetened drink by about 50 percent.[6] If it works for thirsty teenagers, maybe it will work for you.

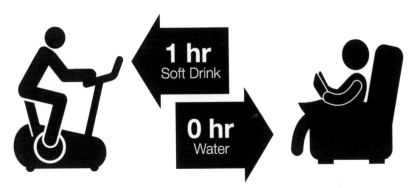

Amount of moderate exercise needed to burn the calories in a 20-ounce (591-mL) sugary soft drink or a glass of water

When you are tempted by junk food, make a rough estimate of the exercise cost, and then ask yourself if the pleasure of eating the food would be worth it. It your answer is yes, commit to the extra exercise *before* you take the first bite. If you have junk food in the house, you can also use a marker to write your best guess of the exercise cost on each package.

You can use an exercise calculator to find the exercise cost of eating junk food. To find an online exercise calculator, search for *calories burned calculator*. Look on the food package to see how many calories it contains. Then use the exercise calculator to figure out how many minutes of your favorite exercise it would take to burn that many calories.

Say You're Not Interested

When it comes to addiction, curiosity is often the last demon to overcome. You tell yourself that you need to take a bite of a tempting food just to see what it tastes like. Then, after one bite, you lose all control and eat the whole thing. This tool targets the curiosity demon directly.

When temptation calls, give it the same response you would a pesky salesman on your doorstep: "I'm not interested." If it keeps talking, repeat the same response, a hundred times if necessary, until it stops: "I'm not interested. I'm not interested. I'm not interested. I'm not interested." Eventually the message will get through to the part of your brain producing the craving, and it will quiet down.

Positive Spin

If politicians can use it, you can, too. Instead of letting temptations get you down, tell yourself that they are simply opportunities to weigh less. When you are tempted to eat a cookie, say to yourself, "If I don't eat that cookie, I will weigh less. What an opportunity!" It *is* true that if you don't eat a cookie, you will weigh less than you would weigh if you did eat it. Reminding yourself of this in a *positive* way can help you say no to temptation without feeling sorry for yourself.

Mindfully Accept the Craving

Mindful acceptance is being aware of your own thoughts and desires (including your cravings) without taking them too seriously, judging them, feeling guilty about them, or reacting to them in an automatic or habitual way.[9,10] Mindfully accepting a craving does not mean that you are happy about it, but only that you see it and accept it for what it is: a natural occurrence that will soon pass, is not a cause for concern, and does not require a response.[11] As you take them less personally and less seriously, the psychological power of your cravings will diminish, and your ability to make calm, rational food decisions will increase.

So how do you develop a mindfully accepting attitude toward your food cravings? Whenever you feel a craving coming on, use the

RAD (Recognize, Accept, Defuse) method to mindfully accept it. The RAD method helps you notice a craving and accept it without giving in to it. There are three steps:

1. Recognize—"I'm having a craving."

2. Accept—"It's OK. It's natural and nothing to feel guilty about. It doesn't mean I'm hungry."

3. Defuse—"It's only a passing emotion. I don't have to follow it."

When you finish step three, go back to step one, and start again. Keep this up for at least a minute, or until the craving is gone. You may want to write these three steps on a card to carry with you as a reminder. See the sample wallet-sized card at the end of this chapter.

Take a Brisk Walk

Scientists at the University of Exeter conducted a pair of experiments that demonstrated a brisk walk can make chocolate less tempting. In one experiment, they instructed a group of chocolate lovers to either take a brisk walk or rest for fifteen minutes before beginning work. The chocolate lovers were then allowed to snack on as much chocolate as they wanted while working. Those who had taken the walk ate only half as much chocolate as those who had rested instead.[7] In the other experiment, a fifteen-minute walk was found to significantly reduce chocolate cravings.[8] If it works for chocolate, it should work for just about anything!

At the first sign of a craving, stand up and head for the door. If brisk walking isn't convenient, try a different exercise. Be sure to exercise with enough intensity that your heart rate increases. If you can't spare fifteen minutes for exercise, do ten minutes or even just five. When you finish, focus your mind on something else.

Also try this technique as a preventive measure. Take a brisk fifteen-minute walk *before* your usual craving time.

This technique not only calms your cravings, but also gives you the added benefit of burning calories and improving your emotional well-being. Using it four times a day would give you a well-spent hour of fat-burning, mood-enhancing, craving-reducing exercise. What tool can beat that?

Getting Started

The biggest step in calming your cravings is the first one: learning a technique that works for you. Different techniques for calming cravings are effective for different people.[12] For the best results, try all of the techniques outlined in this chapter a few times to see which ones are most helpful.

 QuickStart Tip—*Take a few minutes to practice one or more of these techniques so you are ready for the next time you have a craving.*

How to Keep a Slip from Becoming a Binge

It's important not only to mindfully accept your cravings but also your occasional failures to resist them. If you give in to a craving and then feel guilty or hopeless, you may end up eating more junk food just to help yourself feel better or because you have given up trying.

Remind yourself that nobody is perfect, making mistakes is normal, and your slip was not the end of the world. Instead of beating yourself up over it, change direction. Every second that passes is a chance to begin to recover from your mistake. It's never too late to do the right thing.

First, limit the damage—stop eating the craved food. Giving in to a craving doesn't have to turn into a binge. It's never easy to stop eating something you've been craving. It can be as though you're on a highway going fast in the wrong direction. What you need to do is slow down and look for an exit.

It's never too late to do the right thing.

Here's a trick that may help you stop eating after you have given in to a craving. As soon as possible, curl the toes of one foot and repeat to yourself, "I am exiting now," or, "I don't really want to eat this." The discomfort of your curled toes and the irony of your self-talk will help anchor you to reality. Keep repeating the phrase and keep your toes curled until you have the presence of mind to stop eating. Then immediately use one of the tools from the previous section to calm your craving.

Second, evaluate what went wrong and make a plan for next time so you won't make the same mistake again. Rehearse your plan a time or two before you are tempted again.

Self-Therapy for Cravings

Does chocolate sing to you? Do you hear a symphony whenever you walk past the candy aisle of a grocery store? Do cookies scream your name? You will probably always be tempted by the foods you crave most, but there is a way to turn down the volume of those temptations.

The basic approach is to calm your emotional reaction to thoughts of the foods you most often crave. You want to make those foods less exciting, or even boring, to think about, so your thoughts are less likely to trigger cravings. Here's how you would use self-therapy to treat an addiction to chocolate chip cookies. You can use the same steps for any food you find particularly tempting:

1. Visualize chocolate chip cookies in a situation that you frequently find tempting. This might be, for example, a plate of cookies that a coworker has brought to the office to share.

2. To this mental image, add one thing that would make the cookies less desirable. This might be a hair sticking out of one of the cookies, or a bit of mold. Keep your visualization realistic and don't be overly dramatic. Your objective is to make the cookies boring, not disturbing; less emotionally arousing, not more. Also, imagine only one negative thing at a time. It's important to keep the mental image simple.

3. Hold this mental image in your mind for a minute or two.

4. Repeat steps one throught three at least twice each day for a week.

5. Whenever you are in a real-life tempting situation with chocolate chip cookies, immediately imagine the hair or mold to make the real cookies less desirable.

Go through this entire process as often as you need to for any food that you find particularly tempting. Each time you do, you are training yourself to think about those foods without getting excited about them. It's the excitement that gets in the way of rational thinking and causes you to give in to temptation.

QuickStart Tip—At fatlossscience.org/book you can find a printable version of the reminder card on the next page. Cut along the outer lines and fold along the inner lines to make a tri-fold, wallet-sized card.

In Case of a Craving

- Focus my thoughts on something else
- Remember what I really want (see below)
- See the food in a different light
- Imagine eating more than I want
- Count the exercise cost
- Say I'm not interested
- Take a brisk walk
- Mindfully accept the craving (see below)

FatLossScience.org

Remember What I Really Want

What do I want more than this food?

Why do I want it?

FatLossScience.org

Mindful Acceptance (RAD)

- Recognize—"I'm having a craving."
- Accept—"It's OK. It's natural and nothing to feel guilty about. It doesn't mean I'm hungry."
- Defuse—"It's only a passing emotion. I don't have to follow it."

Prevent a Binge

- "I'm exiting now." (Curl toes)

FatLossScience.org

5
How It Adds Up

The Simple Math of Weight Loss

Your body burns calories to supply the energy that you need to live, work, and play. If you eat more calories than you need for your daily activities, your body stores the extra calories as fat. As long as you continue eating more calories than you need, your calorie reserves (fat) continue to grow.

The equation below summarizes what happens to the calories in the food you eat. Neither your genetics nor your food environment can change this simple mathematical truth:

$$\textbf{\textit{Calories stored}} = \textit{calories eaten} - \textit{calories burned.}$$

Think of calories as money. If you earn (eat) just a little more than you spend (burn), your savings (fat) will gradually grow over time.

When you eat fewer calories than you need for your daily activities, your body dips into the savings and some of your fat is burned to supply the needed energy. When this happens, you begin to lose weight.[1] Even a small change in your eating or exercise habits, if continued long enough, can make a big difference in your weight over time.

Metabolism Made Easy

Your body burns calories through a process called *metabolism*. Metabolism supplies energy for physical activity, to digest food, to keep your body warm, and for organ function and repair.

The number of calories your body burns each day just for organ function and repair is called your *resting metabolic rate* (RMR). Your RMR is often referred to in casual speech as your *resting metabolism* or simply *metabolism*. This is the number of calories your body would burn in a day if you did nothing but sleep.

Your RMR is mostly determined by how much muscle tissue you have, and how big your organs (heart, liver, brain, etc.) are. The greater the mass of your muscles and organs, the faster your RMR. Body fat also increases your RMR, but to a lesser degree.

Although there are various ways to calculate your RMR, the following simple equation gives a good rough estimate:[2]

$$RMR = \textit{fat-free weight x 10 + 500}$$

For example, if you weigh 160 pounds, and 25 percent of that weight is from fat, then your *fat-free* weight is 120 pounds. You would calculate your RMR like this:

$$RMR = 120 \; x \; 10 + 500 = \textbf{1,700 calories}$$

Thus, you would burn about 1,700 calories (about three cheeseburgers) each day without even getting out of bed. If you weigh yourself in kilograms instead of pounds, replace the *10* with *22* in the above equations.

To calculate your own RMR, you would, of course, need to know your percentage of body fat. Skinfold measurements provide a reasonably accurate way of doing this. The easiest way to take skinfold measurements is with body fat calipers, which can be purchased online and usually come with detailed instructions for calculating percentage of body fat.

My point here, however, is not to advocate calorie counting as a tool for natural weight loss. It is to help you understand the relationship between metabolism and weight loss. Your resting metabolism mostly reflects the amount of organ and muscle tissue you have, and is about the same as the metabolism of the next man or woman who has the same amount of muscle and organ tissue. If that next man or woman seems to have an easier time keeping the weight off than you do, a faster metabolism is probably *not* the reason.

What Makes Your Metabolism Unique?

Women generally have slower RMRs than men, mostly because of their typically smaller frames and less muscle mass. People who are naturally larger framed and muscular have relatively fast RMRs. Thus, the most important genes affecting your metabolism are the ones that influence your frame size and muscle mass.

Having a slower RMR than someone else is not a problem unless you try to eat as much as they do. Your body simply doesn't need as many calories to function.

The RMR of a non-exercising adult typically decreases 2 to 5 percent every decade, mostly due to lack of physical activity and loss of muscle and organ mass. This trend is reversible. You can boost your metabolism at any age with muscle-building exercises.[3]

Losing weight can also decrease your RMR, primarily because when you lose weight, you usually lose some muscle as well as fat, and the lost muscle and fat are no longer using calories. Proper muscle-building exercises during a period of gradual weight loss can help preserve your muscle mass and keep your metabolism up.

You can boost your metabolism at any age with muscle-building exercises.

Your daily activities also affect your metabolism. In addition to the calories burned by resting metabolism, a non-exercising adult will burn about 20 percent more calories each day moving around, digesting food, and maintaining body temperature. A moderately active adult (for example, one who plays an active sport or exercises three to five days a week) will burn a total of about 50 percent more calories.[4]

6
Eat Less
(Without Going Hungry)

Even a small change in the amount of food you eat each day can make a big difference in your weight over time. For example, eating one hundred calories more than you need each day (a very small soft drink or the mayonnaise on a sandwich) can cause you to gain several pounds each year. You can burn off those hundred calories each day by walking briskly for about a half hour (if you weigh about 150 lbs or 70 kg). Alternatively, you can save yourself the trouble by making some minor changes to your eating habits, such as eating your sandwich with mustard instead of mayonnaise, or drinking ice water instead of a sugary soft drink.

We usually don't intend to eat too much. We overeat, often without thinking, because of poor food choices, bad habits, and the temptations around us. In this chapter, you will learn how changes in your food choices, habits, and personal environment can help you eat fewer calories without going hungry.

Eat More Natural Weight Loss Foods

Researchers at Harvard University conducted a study in which they monitored the weight and habits of 120,877 adults over a twenty-year period. They found that study participants who increased their consumption of fruits, nuts, vegetables, whole grains, or yogurt tended to lose weight, while those who decreased their consumption of any of these foods tended to gain weight.[1]

Eating more of these natural weight loss foods can help you lose weight also. Unprocessed fruit, nuts, vegetables, and grains digest relatively slowly because of the fiber they contain and because their tissue structure hasn't already been broken up by processing. Foods that digest slowly reach your blood stream gradually, so you remain satisfied longer after a meal ends.[2] As a result, you are less tempted to snack between meals or overeat during the next one.

It isn't entirely clear why yogurt is associated with weight loss. It may simply be that adding yogurt to a meal makes it more satisfying so you end up eating less overall. Yogurt may also slow the digestion of the meal so you don't get hungry again so soon.

As you eat more fruits, nuts, vegetables, whole grains, and yogurt, reduce the amount of less-healthy foods in your diet by eating them less often and in smaller portions.

Fresh Fruit

In the Harvard study, fruits were associated with weight loss while fruit juices were associated with weight gain. Fresh whole or cut-up fruit is preferable to fruit juices or other processed fruit because it usually has more fiber, digests more slowly, and has fewer calories. A 12-ounce (355-mL) glass of orange juice, for example, has about 170 calories. A medium orange has only 60. Here are some ways to eat more fresh fruit:

- Eat a small handful of nuts and a piece of fruit along with a glass of water for a snack.

- Add a piece of fresh fruit to breakfast, lunch, or dinner.

- Buy a variety of whole, cut-up, and frozen fruit. People tend to eat what they have in the house, so keep your house well-stocked with good food.

- Keep a bowl of fresh fruit on the table.

- Keep a container of cut-up fruit in the refrigerator. To keep the fruit from turning brown, add some lemon juice.

- Add fruit to cereal for breakfast.

- Make a yogurt parfait or dip cut-up fruit in low-fat yogurt for breakfast or a snack. Top a bowl of cut-up fruit with yogurt for an easy dessert.

- Make a fruit salad with grapes or berries and cut-up fruit. Add plain or flavored yogurt if you like it creamy. Top it with shredded coconut or chopped nuts.

- Add cut-up fruit, grapes, berries, orange sections, raisins, or dried cranberries to a green salad.

- If oranges and other acidic fruit make your teeth sensitive, try eating them with yogurt.[3]

Nuts

Although nuts are relatively high in calories, they also contain fiber, fat, and protein, which slow digestion and provide enduring satisfaction. You need only a small handful with a meal or snack to get the weight loss benefits. Because nuts are dry, be sure to eat them with a glass of water to get the full effect. Here are some ways to get more nuts into your diet:

- Buy a large container of nuts and divide them into handful-sized portions. Keep these portions handy to add to packed lunches or snacks.

- Eat a small handful of nuts with breakfast, lunch, or dinner.

- Add nuts to cereal or low-fat yogurt for breakfast.

- Eat a yogurt parfait with nuts as a snack or with a meal.

- Add nuts to green salads, vegetable dishes, and fruit salads.

Vegetables

The US government's *Dietary Guidelines for Americans 2010* recommends that half of the food on your plate be fruits and vegetables.[4] Here are some ways to eat more vegetables:

- Stock up on frozen vegetables for simple, fast side dishes.

- Keep a container of baby carrots, celery sticks, sliced green peppers or cucumber, or other ready-to-eat vegetables in a see-through container in the refrigerator for lunches and snacks. Put carrots and celery sticks in a container of water so they stay crisp.

- If you don't care for vegetables, eat them when you are hungriest so they will taste better, and you will gradually learn to enjoy them more.

- Add cut-up vegetables to a packed lunch, or take some along to add to a purchased lunch.

- Add vegetables prepared two or three different ways (cut-up raw, steamed, roasted, etc.) to dinner.

- Sprinkle cooked vegetables with feta, Parmesan, vinegar, or other strong flavors to make them more interesting.

- Include a green salad and low-calorie dressing with dinner every evening.

- Try a large green salad topped with sliced boiled eggs or chicken breast for lunch.

- Try low-fat yogurt seasoned with dill weed, mint, or other herbs as a dip for cut vegetables.

- Top fried or scrambled eggs with tomato salsa, nopales, or fresh avocado.

- Decorate dinner plates with vegetable slices.

- Add grated or chopped vegetables to some of your usual recipes. Zucchini, carrots, tomatoes, and spinach can be added to many dishes.

- Add steamed vegetables to soups.

- When you eat out, request additional vegetables. For example, ask for extra tomatoes, pickles, or lettuce on a sandwich, or extra vegetable toppings on a pizza.

- Grill vegetables such as onions, mushrooms, and green peppers as part of a barbeque meal.

See appendix A for some easy vegetable recipes. The recipes in this book are custom-made for people who don't like to cook, or who like to cook but don't have much time. Each has only a few ingredients and requires minimal cooking skills. With them, you can quickly make simple dishes that you won't soon tire of and that will help you lose weight.

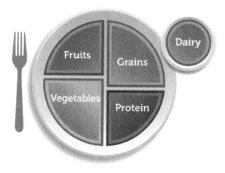

Recommended proportions of food groups in a meal (US Department of Agriculture, ChooseMyPlate.gov)

Whole and Slowly-Digesting Grains

A whole grain is a grain that still has the bran and germ. The bran of a grain is the outer, high-fiber layer. The germ is the high-fat, high-protein embryo of the grain plant. A *refined* grain has the bran and germ removed. *Processing* refers to any alteration of a grain, including removal of the bran and germ in the refining process, grinding of grain into flour, bleaching of flour, or treatment of a grain so it cooks more quickly.

Unlike the minimally processed grain eaten by our ancestors, most of the grain in the modern diet is in a highly processed form—much of it as refined flour. The process of converting wheat to refined flour increases its caloric density by over 10 percent, reduces its fiber content by about 80 percent, and reduces its protein content by almost 30 percent.[5]

The less processing a grain goes through before you eat it, the more slowly it digests, so it keeps you satisfied longer and you don't get hungry so soon. Because flour is ground so finely and is so low in fiber, fat, and protein, it digests very quickly. Whole wheat flour is better, but still digests rather quickly if it is finely ground. Food products made of coarsely ground flour digest more slowly because of the extra time required for breaking down the larger particles.[6,7] Food products with a high proportion of cracked, sprouted, or intact grains digest even more slowly.[8] Brown rice generally digests more slowly than white rice.

Besides differences in levels of processing, differences in the grains themselves affect the rate of digestion. For example, high-amylose varieties of rice, such as basmati, digest more slowly than low amylose varieties. Low amylose rice tends to be sticky and digests rather quickly, whether it is white or brown. Converted rice digests slowly, even though it's not brown. Genuine rye bread digests more slowly than wheat bread.[9] Pasta made of semolina digests more slowly than other pasta and most bread. Pasta cooked *al dente*, meaning that it is still firm, digests more slowly than pasta that is overcooked.

When shopping for whole grain products, check the list of ingredients. Whole grain foods usually have one of the following as the first ingredient: brown rice, buckwheat, bulgur, millet, oatmeal, quinoa, rolled oats, whole-grain barley, whole-grain corn, whole-grain sorghum, whole-grain triticale, whole oats, whole rye, whole wheat, or wild rice. The following usually do *not* indicate whole-grain ingredients: wheat flour, wheat, stone-ground, multigrain, and 100% wheat. Here are some ways to eat more slowly-digesting grains:

- For breakfast, eat hot cereal made of a minimally processed grain such as flaked or cracked wheat, old-fashioned rolled oats, steel-cut oats, bulgur, quinoa, brown basmati rice, or hulled millet. To save time, cook up a large batch and warm a portion in the microwave for breakfast every day. If you prefer cold cereal, try the granola recipe in appendix B.

- Use brown basmati rice, bulgur, hulled millet, or quinoa in a side dish recipe for dinner.

- When you eat out, request whole grain options. For example, request brown rice instead of white rice, or whole wheat bread instead of white bread.

- Buy bread made of whole grains or, even better, of sprouted or cracked grains.

- Buy semolina pasta, and cook it al dente.

- Use whole grain flour or oatmeal for some or all of the flour in pancakes, waffles, cookies, bread, muffins, scones, and other flour-based recipes.

- For baking, try medium-ground whole cornmeal, coarse or medium ground whole wheat flour, whole spelt flour, or whole rye flour. Look for these products in the natural foods section of your grocery store or in a health food store.

- Buy a portable home mill and grind your own flour, using a coarse setting.

See appendix B for some easy grain recipes.

Yogurt

Yogurt in your meal will make it more satisfying. Yogurt also makes a quick, satisfying snack. Plain low-fat yogurt has relatively few calories.

As with most any habit, the hardest part of adding yogurt to your snacks and meals is just getting started. We tend to eat what we have on hand, so buy a quart or two of plain low-fat yogurt as well as some ready-to-eat portions of your favorite flavored low-fat, low-sugar yogurt, and put them in your refrigerator. Here are some more ideas:

- Make a yogurt parfait for breakfast or a snack by mixing plain yogurt with fruit and granola or whole-grain breakfast cereal.

- Eat plain yogurt as a topping in place of sour cream on just about any hot dish. Try it on vegetables.

- Mix plain yogurt into your favorite salad dressing to make it lower-calorie.

- Use plain Greek yogurt in recipes in place of sour cream or cream cheese.

- Eat yogurt as a lunch or dinner side dish.

- Enjoy yogurt sweetened with a little jam or honey in place of less healthy desserts.

See appendix C for some easy yogurt recipes.

Eat a Solid Breakfast, Lunch, and Dinner

Skipped or unbalanced meals can leave you hungry or unsatisfied and tempted to snack on junk food or overeat later in the day.

In a balanced meal, according to the *Dietary Guidelines for Americans 2010*, about half (45–65 percent) of the calories are from carbohydrates and the remainder are split between protein (10–35 percent) and fat (20–35 percent).[4] Keeping each meal within the recommended ranges for carbohydrates, protein, and fat will help keep you satisfied between meals. While the carbohydrates will help you feel satisfied quickly, the fats, proteins, and fiber will serve to slow the digestion of the meal so that you don't get hungry so soon.[10,11] A combination of carbohydrates, fat, and protein will also help your body get the nutrients and constant supply of energy it needs for good health and calorie-burning physical activities.

The carbohydrate portion of a meal should consist mostly of minimally processed vegetables, beans, and whole grains.

The protein portion of a meal should come from nuts, beans, soy products, eggs, fish, milk products, whole grains, or lean unprocessed meats.

Keep in mind that there are more than twice as many calories in a gram of fat as there are in a gram of protein or carbohydrate. This means that the amount of fat needed for a balanced meal is relatively small. Common sources of fat in a meal include salad dressing, milk, meat, nuts, beans, whole grain, bakery goods, and cooking oil.

The best drink to have with your meal is water. It doesn't add any calories, yet in combination with the fiber in foods it can help you feel full.

A good, solid breakfast is especially important to help prevent hunger and cravings, so you are less tempted to snack on junk food during the day.

A study by scientists at Virginia Commonwealth University and Hospital de Clinicas Caracas in Venezuela found that dieters who ate a moderately-sized breakfast (610 calories of a 1,240 daily calorie diet) each day initially lost less weight than dieters who ate a small breakfast (290 calories of a 1,085 daily calorie diet), but were more successful at keeping the weight off. Although the dieters who ate the small breakfasts lost more weight at first, they gained much of it back before the end of the eight-month study, apparently because they were less successful at resisting food temptations. By the end of the study, dieters who ate the moderately sized breakfasts had lost about four times as much weight as the other group. They also reported less hunger and fewer cravings throughout the day.[12]

A bowl of cold cereal for breakfast isn't enough. Instead, try to include a whole grain, some unprocessed fruit or vegetables, and a protein source such as eggs, nuts, or low-fat yogurt. Make up for those extra breakfast calories by snacking less or by eating less at dinner, then go to bed before you start to get hungry again. You need more calories in the morning for energy and insurance against food temptations, and fewer in the evening when you are relaxing or about to go to bed.

Eat Less Junk Food

Eat less of refined-floury and sugary foods, potato-based foods, white rice, high-calorie dressings and toppings, and sugary and alcoholic drinks. These are the common junk foods of the modern western diet. You can cut back on these foods without feeling hungry if you eat more of the natural weight loss foods discussed previously.

Refined-Floury and Sugary Foods

Most processed foods have been "predigested" to a degree during grinding, juicing, or other processing, so they digest rather quickly, leaving you with a load of calories and a soon-empty stomach. Processed foods high in refined flour or added sugar, such as bread, candy, cold breakfast cereals, cookies, cake, doughnuts, pancakes, pastries, pizza, and waffles are not only implicated in the weight gain epidemic, but also in the recent dramatic increase in diabetes.[13]

Refined flour is any flour that is not whole grain. Sugars commonly added to food include sucrose, maltose, glucose, fructose, brown sugar, molasses, honey, maple syrup, agave nectar, corn syrup, raw sugar, and corn sweetener. Any of these added sugars will contribute to weight gain, no matter how "natural" they are. Refined flour and added sugar provide energy (i.e., calories), but little in the way of nutrients. If you are overweight, you are already consuming too much energy. Refined flour and sugar also encourage overeating by enhancing the flavor of foods to an unnatural degree. Here are some ways to eat less of these foods:

- Buy bread made of sprouted grain instead of flour.

- Beware of ready-to-eat breakfast foods that are high in sugar and refined flour. For a better breakfast, try whole grain hot cereal or toasted bread made of sprouted grain. Avoid cold breakfast cereals unless they are unsweetened and made of whole grains.

- Set reasonable limits. You don't need to eliminate desserts and other sweets entirely. Allowing yourself one small dessert a day, with more allowed on special occasions, can help keep your spirits up and decrease the temptation to cheat.

- If you have an urge for something sweet, eat fruit.

- When you eat pasta, make sure it is semolina or whole grain, and cooked al dente.

- When you buy a burger, discard half of the bun. Eat sandwiches open-face.

- Read the ingredients on food packages. Any food that has refined flour or an added sugar as the first ingredient should be eaten sparingly.

- Prepare your own meals. At least you will know what's in them.

- Have plenty of fruits or vegetables in each meal. Filling your stomach with these relatively low-calorie foods will help you feel satisfied without eating so much of the higher-calorie foods.

- Have a light (not creamy) soup with lunch or dinner. This will slow down your eating, giving your stomach more time to produce feelings of satisfaction.

- Don't shop when you are hungry, and decide ahead of time what you will buy.

- Decide what you will have for each meal a day in advance so that you are not left deciding what to eat when you are already hungry. Write your decisions down. Prepare meals ahead of time, when possible, to further limit last-minute decisions.

Potato-based Foods

A few unprocessed foods, such as potatoes, digest quickly. Potatoes with added fat, such as french fries, hash browns, and potato chips, digest more slowly but are much higher in calories. In the Harvard study,[1] potato-based foods had a greater association with weight gain than any other food category. Here are some ways to eat less of potato-based foods:

- At a restaurant, order a side salad, low-fat yogurt, or fresh fruit instead of fries. Skipping the fries can save you the trouble of having to work off 350 to 400 extra calories (for a medium order).

- Substitute sweet potatoes, parsnips, carrots, turnips, or other vegetables for regular potatoes in your meals.

- Snack on fresh fruit, celery sticks, or baby carrots instead of potato chips.

- Avoid temptation by keeping potato chips and other potato-based snack foods out of the house.

White Rice

White rice has had the outer layers and the germ of the grain removed. What is left is mostly starch, which digests directly to sugar. White rice digests quite quickly, especially if it is sticky (low amylose), leaving you with a load of calories but little lasting satisfaction.

To eat less white rice, try substituting brown basmati rice or converted rice. If you don't like the flavor of brown rice, try adding a little lemon juice.

High-Calorie Dressings and Toppings

Salad dressings, mayonnaise, butter, and sour cream pack a lot of calories in a little space. Having some fat in your meal is important, but don't overdo it.

It makes no sense to pour 300 calories of dressing on a 30-calorie salad. Almost all of the calories are coming from the dressing. If you cut the amount of dressing in half, you will reduce the total calories you are eating by almost half. Here are some more ways to eat less of high-calorie dressings and toppings:

- When you order a salad, get dressing on the side so you can take just what you need. When eating at home, make your favorite salad dressing lighter by mixing it with plain low-fat yogurt.

- When you order a burger or sandwich, request it with only a little mayonnaise, or with mustard instead.

- Buy low-fat dressings or make your own. See appendix C for salad dressing recipes using low-fat yogurt.

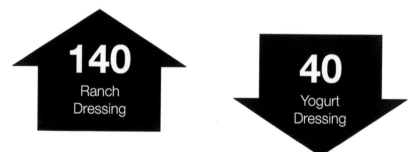

Calories in 2 tablespoons (30 mL) of regular ranch dressing or low-fat yogurt dressing

Sugary and Alcoholic Drinks

Sugary and alcoholic drinks are high in calories and low in nutrients. Drinking calories is a fast way to gain body fat because you can ingest hundreds of calories in just a few minutes. *Dietary Guidelines for Americans 2010* recommends careful monitoring of sugar-sweetened drinks, fruit juices, and alcoholic drinks, because they are high in calories and easily over consumed.[4]

Water is the only drink the human body requires, and is needed in generous amounts for optimal body function and weight loss. Water has no calories and won't spark your appetite like other drinks can. Here are some ways to cut down on liquid calories:

- Don't have high-calorie drinks in your house where they can tempt you. Stick with water or low-calorie drinks such as tea without sugar. Most sports drinks are high-calorie.

- Drink water when you are feeling hungry or thirsty between meals.

- Fruit juices are high-calorie. Eat fresh fruit instead.

- When you eat out, request ice water or a low-calorie drink instead of a sugary soft drink to avoid having to work off about 150 calories or more (for a small soft drink).

- If you don't like the flavor of plain water, add a squeeze of lemon juice.

The Power of Half

If you don't want to entirely eliminate some of these junk foods, a good goal might be to eat them half as often as you now do, and in portions half the usual size. This approach won't leave you feeling deprived, but will greatly decrease your calorie intake. Eating half as much, half as often, will reduce your consumption of these foods—and their calories—by a full 75 percent. That's a lot of calories you won't have to burn.

 QuickStart Tip—*Write down the junk foods you eat most often. Using the suggestions in this chapter, the recipes in the back of the book, and your own ideas, list some healthy foods you could substitute.*

Eat Junk Food Only with Meals

Eat junk food only as part of a meal. Drink only water between meals. For snacks, eat fruit, nuts, vegetables, minimally processed grains, or low-fat yogurt. You will be less likely to overeat when snacking on healthy, unprocessed foods, and they will keep you satisfied longer. If you eat solid, balanced meals, you won't get as hungry between meals and may not need to snack at all.

Water is the only drink the human body requires.

Junk foods tend to be nutritionally unbalanced and highly processed. As a result, they tend to digest rather quickly, leaving you soon hungry. Eating your junk food with an otherwise healthy meal will help you eat less of it. The other foods in the meal will also help buffer the effects of the junk food on your blood sugar levels, so you remain satisfied longer after the meal ends and are less likely to experience cravings later in the day.

Eat Mindfully

Mindfulness, remember, means paying attention to your present experience. Mindful eating means keeping your attention focused on what and how much you are eating. It is the opposite of mindless eating, which is what most people do most of the time. When you eat mindlessly, you put food in your mouth because it's there, not because you need it or necessarily even want it. Mindful eating will not only enable you to get greater enjoyment from a smaller amount of food, but will also give your body more time to feel satisfied so you are less tempted to overeat. There are five steps to mindful eating:

1. Decide how much you will eat before you start. Remember, if you eat foods that digest more slowly and that provide more nutrients, you don't have to eat as much each meal to avoid feeling hungry before the next one. Most fruits and vegetables don't contain many calories, so they can be eaten in greater quantities than other foods. Put everything you plan to eat on your plate, then put away or discard the remainder.

2. Avoid distracting influences. Don't watch television or read while eating. We tend to keep eating until the end of the story, whether we are hungry or not.

3. Take and savor little bites. Much of our eating is not out of hunger but to enjoy the flavors and textures of our favorite foods. You can eat less while enjoying it just as much, if you eat slowly and deliberately. Take small bites and consciously savor each one, making a point to hold the food in your mouth a little longer and notice the textures and flavors. After a while your taste buds will begin to tire of the flavor, and you will be less tempted to overeat.

4. Put your fork or spoon down or take a small sip of water between bites. This will slow your eating down, giving your stomach time to produce feelings of fullness and satisfaction and allowing you to pay better attention to those feelings.

5. Listen to your stomach. When empty, your stomach is about the size of your fist. It only holds a couple of handfuls of food comfortably. If you eat more than that, it stretches to the point that it begins to put pressure on other organs. Let the feeling of your stomach rather than the flavor of the food tell you how much to eat. Stop eating when your stomach feels a little heavy. If it feels tight, stretched, or topped off, you've had too much. Don't feel that you have to finish all of your food. Your mother was wrong. It's OK to leave food on your plate, especially if you have been served too much. Don't treat yourself like a garbage disposal just to get rid of extra food.

Limit Restaurant Meals

Limit fast food and restaurant dining. Restaurants are generally focused on making food that tastes good, not that is good for you. The sugar, fats, and refined carbohydrates they use to make the food highly palatable also make it high-calorie. Also, the sizes of restaurant meals have increased in recent decades to the point that they are often enough for two or more people. Since our natural tendency is to keep eating until the portion in front of us is gone, we end up eating too much.[14] Here are some ways to eat less restaurant food:

- Take a few minutes to prepare a meal and take it with you instead of eating out.

- When eating at a restaurant, select small or mini options when available. Regular sized portions these days are already "super sized" compared to portions twenty or thirty years ago.[15] A "bargain" isn't a bargain when it's more than you want or need. The first few bites of anything usually taste the best anyway.

- Split a meal with a companion, or ask for a box before you start eating and put aside part of the meal to take home.

- Don't feel that you have to finish your food. Getting your "money's worth" by finishing your meal doesn't make much sense when you consider the medical and lifestyle costs of obesity-related diseases or the time and effort you'll need to burn off the extra calories.

- Eat at home when you can. Use some of the simple recipes from the appendices at the back of this book to make quick, healthy meals.

Get Enough Sleep

Studies have found that sleeping less than six or seven hours a night is a risk factor for becoming obese. This may be partly due to the role of sleep in determining the levels of hormones that control hunger.[16] Here are some ways to get more and better sleep:

- Plan your bedtime before it gets close. Don't arrive at home without a plan.

- Try to arrange your schedule so you can get to bed at about the same time every night, even on weekends. It will be easier to turn bedtime into a habit if it's at a consistent time.

- Don't go to bed hungry, or full. Eating close to bedtime can disrupt sleep, but being too hungry can make you restless also. Eat a solid dinner and then go to bed before you get hungry again.

- Avoid caffeine, alcohol, and nicotine in the evening. If you are having trouble falling asleep or sleeping soundly, any of these substances might be to blame.

- Exercise. Exercising regularly can help you sleep better. Exercising in the evening, however, may make it harder to fall asleep.

- Keep it cool and dark. Warmth and light signal daytime and wakefulness to your body. Cool and dark signal night and sleep.

- Keep pets and kids out of the bed. The extra wiggles make sleep more difficult.

- Relax your mind. Going to bed with heavy thoughts makes it more difficult to fall asleep, and to sleep soundly. Avoid television, computer work, intense reading, or anything else that overly engages your thoughts or emotions before bedtime. Use meditation, light stretching, a warm bath, or another relaxing activity to leave behind the worries of the day. Make a list of things to think about the next day, then forget about them and go to sleep.

Watch Less Television

Television takes time away from sleep and physical activity. It leaves less time for preparing meals, so you are more likely to eat unhealthy prepared foods. Television viewing also encourages snacking on junk food. Many calories are eaten and few are burned in front of the television.

Not surprisingly, television watching was associated with weight gain in the Harvard study.[1] People who spend a lot of time watching television are more likely to be overweight than moderate viewers or non-viewers. A study of over fourteen hundred successful weight loss maintainers revealed that most watched ten or fewer hours of television per week, compared to the US national average of twenty-eight hours of television viewing for adults.[17]

Television can be addictive, so cutting back may be difficult at first, but with time other activities will become more enjoyable and television will seem less important.[18]

Many calories are eaten and few are burned in front of the television.

Turn off the television and fill your leisure time with activities that burn calories and that make snacking less convenient. Here are some ways to watch less television:

- Plan your weekly television schedule ahead of time, and then stick with it.

- Fill your week with productive activities so you won't have time to watch television. Plan activities ahead of time. Don't arrive home without a plan.

- Don't leave the television turned on when no one is watching it. If silence is unbearable, play music or turn on the radio.

- Unplug your television or cover it when it isn't being used. Attach a note to the cover listing several things you could be doing instead of watching television—meditating, exercising, playing catch with a child, enjoying a hobby, learning a new skill, visiting with a friend.

- Put remotes out of easy reach.

- Don't turn the television on because you are bored or just to see what's on. Find another cure for boredom.

- Remove television sets from bedrooms and eating areas.

Many of these ideas also apply to other time-burners such as recreational Internet use, video games, and videos.

 QuickStart Tip—*Take a minute to decide on one thing you can do to watch less television. Write it down and commit to doing it.*

7
Be Active
(Without Wasting Time)

The human body is designed to be moving and working throughout the day. Sitting for long periods in an automobile, at a desk, or on a couch is an unnatural situation. It should not be surprising, then, that regular physical activity has many potential health benefits. These include better cognitive function; improved sleep quality; healthier bones and joints; greater muscle strength and endurance; and lower risks of depression, heart disease, stroke, metabolic syndrome, high blood pressure, diabetes, osteoporosis, and some cancers. It is also important for maintaining a healthy weight.[1]

Regular exercise isn't required for losing weight; just about any diet will do that. Regular exercise is needed to keep the weight off. The National Weight Loss Registry is a long-term study of individuals who have lost thirty or more pounds and kept it off for at least a year. To maintain their weight loss, registry members report burning about 370 calories per day by exercising. This equates to about thirty-five to forty-five minutes of vigorous exercise or sixty to seventy-five minutes of moderate exercise.[2] These numbers are only averages. You may be able to get by with less, especially if you make use of much of the other advice in this book. It is unlikely, however, that you will be able to lose weight and keep it off without a regular exercise program.

Regular exercise is needed to keep the weight off.

The US government's *2008 Physical Activity Guidelines for Americans* recommends at least thirty minutes of moderate exercise five or more days a week for basic health, and suggests that sixty or more minutes a day may be needed to reach or maintain a healthy body weight. The daily exercise may be done all at once or divided into smaller blocks, but each block should be a minimum of ten minutes. Fifteen minutes of vigorous exercise may be substituted for every thirty minutes of moderate exercise.[1]

Turn Work and Play into Exercise

Getting thirty minutes of moderate exercise each day can be as simple as taking a brisk walk when you get up in the morning or during your lunch hour. Other moderate exercise options include hiking, light weight training or calisthenics, yoga, shooting baskets, recreational swimming, bicycling, or playing actively with children. Vigorous exercise might include racquetball, basketball, doubles tennis, running or jogging, fast ballroom or square dancing, fast bicycling, skiing, hiking hills, swimming laps, jumping rope, or heavy weight training.[1] Find an activity that you enjoy. Staying with an exercise program is easier if you make it fun. See the list at the end of chapter 8 for ideas for making your exercise program a success. Here are some more ways to be active:

- Join an exercise group.

- Get a gym membership and use it.

- Organize a group of friends or neighbors for morning or evening walks.

- Take stairs instead of elevators.

- Walk instead of drive, or park a distance from your destination and walk the rest of the way.

Get Away from the Screen

Limit television and other leisure screen time such as videos and recreational Internet use. These activities take time away from active recreation, burn very few calories, and leave you feeling less energetic.

Limiting leisure screen time to a few hours a week can facilitate your efforts to get more physical activity. Getting away from the screen and living an active life is also kind of like starring in your own reality show. Enjoy it!

To cut down on your leisure screen time, try some of the suggestions for watching less television at the end of chapter 6.

 QuickStart Tip—Take a minute to write down some ideas for calorie-burning activities to do on a daily or weekly basis.

8
Boost Your Metabolism
(Without Drugs)

Endurance exercises such as fast walking, biking, swimming, and running can increase your total daily metabolism by burning calories directly, by increasing your resting metabolic rate (RMR),[1,2] and by boosting your energy levels so you are more inclined to do other physical activities.

Strength-building exercises can have an even greater effect on RMR by adding muscle mass.[3] They can replace muscle lost due to physical inactivity and also help prevent additional muscle loss as you eat fewer daily calories.[4]

Keep in mind that a given volume of muscle weighs more than the same volume of fat. This means that if you are building muscle at the same time you are losing fat, you may become more slender without actually losing much weight.

Some women worry that strength training will make them look bulky. It will not unless they have very unusual genetics.[5] Instead, strength training can help support a pleasing posture and add muscle tone and definition for a more slender and attractive appearance.

Strengthening exercises can provide you with many health benefits at any age, but particularly as you get older. Properly conducted strength training can be a virtual Fountain of Youth by increasing muscle mass, metabolic rate, and bone density and by reducing body fat, resting blood pressure, low back pain, arthritic pain, depression, and age-related muscle loss. It can also improve glucose metabolism, which is important for those with type 2 diabetes.[6,7]

Properly conducted strength training can be a virtual Fountain of Youth.

You don't need weights or any special equipment to strength train. Push-ups, arm and leg lifts, bridges, planks, abdominal curls, and other body-weight exercises will take you a long way.[8] Choose a combination of exercises that work all your major muscle groups, including your core abdominal muscles.

To avoid injury, start easy and increase the intensity of your exercises gradually so your body has a chance to adjust to each new exercise. Be sure to warm up before each exercise session and to use proper form. For most exercises, proper form includes keeping your abs tight and your back straight, with a slight inward curve in your lower back. One way to warm up is to begin each exercise by doing several repetitions with about half the weight that you normally lift. If you are doing a body-weight exercise instead of lifting weights, warm up by first doing several repetitions of an easier version of the exercise. For example, do some pushups on your knees before beginning pushups on your toes.

Strength train two or three days a week, leaving at least one day between each exercise day for your muscles to recover.[9] Choose a time of day to exercise when you are most energetic so you can work your muscles harder.

If you are lifting weights, use weights that are light enough that you can do at least eight repetitions of an exercise in proper form.[10] Stay at that weight until you can do twelve or more repetitions of the exercise for two consecutive exercise days. Then you can add about 5 percent more weight the next day you exercise. Be sure to perform each repetition of an exercise slowly and smoothly through a full range of motion, taking at least six full seconds to complete it. One set of each exercise is enough as long as it thoroughly fatigues your muscles.[11]

After completing each exercise, stretch the target muscles for twenty or thirty seconds to promote muscle development and flexibility.[12] Breathe normally during the stretch. To avoid injury, move slowly, and stretch only to the point where you feel a moderate stretching sensation. Stretching should not be painful.

Consult your doctor before beginning an intensive exercise program, and get proper training before working with heavy weights or doing unfamiliar exercises.

For many, the hardest part of an exercise program is getting started. Here are some ideas for getting started with, and consistently following, a strengthening exercise program:

- Schedule two or three times a week for strengthening exercises.
- Write your exercise schedule on a piece of paper and put it where you will see it every day. Even better, put it where you will have to move it every day, such as on your car seat or kitchen table.

- Choose three or four exercises to begin with. You can add more or try different ones later. There are many excellent exercise websites, magazines, and books that can give you ideas and teach you proper exercise techniques. If you haven't done strengthening exercises for a while, start with some easy ones.

- Commit to spend at least five minutes exercising during your scheduled time, even if you don't feel like it. Chances are that after five minutes, you will feel motivated enough to continue and complete your session.

- Have a backup plan to do a simpler exercise session if you are unable to do your regularly scheduled one. For example, if your basic plan is to exercise at a gym, have a backup plan to do some bodyweight exercises at home for a few minutes if you can't make it to the gym.

- If you miss an exercise session, don't give up or beat yourself up over it. Just commit to make your next one.

- Lay your exercise clothes out the night before your scheduled exercise session so they are ready and waiting for you.

- Exercise with a friend. Agreeing to exercise with another person can make a big difference in your motivation. If you can't find a partner to exercise with, join an exercise group or hire a personal trainer.

- Hold yourself accountable for following through with your exercise sessions. There are different ways to do this. You can make a commitment to report regularly on a fitness web site, on your own Internet blog, or to a friend. Another option is to create a monthly chart to fill in as you complete each exercise session.

▪ Reward yourself at the end of the month if you have met your goals. Don't require perfection of yourself, but choose a realistic goal to call success. For example, completing at least two out of three sessions each week for a month may be a good enough goal to start with.

 QuickStart Tip—*Think of a friend who might be willing to exercise with you, or even to just set exercise goals with you. Call or send a message to your friend to get started.*

9
Myths

When it comes to weight loss advice, myths abound, and distinguishing fact from fallacy can be difficult. It helps that many weight loss myths have been the subjects of scientific studies. Here are a few common myths, along with the facts.

"People who have difficulty controlling their weight often have naturally slow metabolisms."

Although some earlier scientific studies incorrectly reached this conclusion,[1] more recent and better-designed studies have generally found that obesity-prone individuals have resting metabolic rates as fast as those of other people with similar muscle and organ mass.[1,2] Studies show that even in infancy and youth, excess weight gain generally results from excess eating rather than slow resting metabolism.[3,4] The faulty conclusions of the earlier studies were at least partially due to the tendency of overweight study participants to underestimate the number of calories they consume by 20 to 50 percent.[5,6,7]

Gaining weight actually increases your metabolic rate. When you gain much fat, you usually gain some extra muscle as well to help move the extra weight around. Both the extra muscle and fat increase your RMR, and more energy is required to move a bigger body. If you are overweight, therefore, you probably have a faster metabolic rate than people of similar frame size who are not overweight. This increase in metabolic rate works against additional weight gain and stabilizes your weight unless you eat even more daily calories than before.

"Some people are genetically fat."

In fact, we are all "genetically fat" when we are in a fattening food environment and live a physically inactive lifestyle. Just as a squirrel is genetically programmed to pack away nuts when they are available in order to survive a hard winter, we are genetically programmed to pack on fat when surrounded by high-calorie, highly palatable food in order to survive times of food scarcity. Weight gain under such conditions is the result of normal genes functioning correctly.[8] The only problem is, the highly palatable food is always around us, and the slimming times of food scarcity never come. If squirrels were always surrounded by nuts they would be overweight too.

We are all "genetically fat" when we are in a fattening food environment and living a physically inactive lifestyle.

Our food environment and lifestyles are broken, not our genes. The modern fattening food environment is very different from the food environment that existed through most of human history. It is far from natural, and combined with a less-active lifestyle, it promotes weight gain for almost anyone who doesn't actively resist it.[9]

The Pima group of American Indians are believed to be genetically fine-tuned for conserving calories. Even this group, however, should not be considered naturally fat. While the Pima living in the United States are one of the most overweight populations in the world, the Pima living in remote regions of Mexico, where the environment is physically demanding and more traditional foods are eaten, are lean like non-Pima Mexicans living in the same environment.[10]

Scientists have found only a few genetic defects that influence body fat enough to be noticeable on an individual basis. These genetic defects are rare and generally act by increasing your tendency to overeat, most often through their effects on hormones that control appetite.[11] There is little evidence for major genetic defects that cause weight gain by slowing metabolism.[12]

Although your individual genetics may make weight loss more difficult, no gene can stop you from losing weight if you are eating fewer calories than you burn. For almost all of us, the genes that are causing most of our weight gain are our normal genes, not our defective ones. We all have genes that are designed to store extra calories as fat. The best way to prevent your genes from causing weight gain is to make your personal environment less fattening and to become more physically active.[13]

"Some people are naturally plump and rounded."

Although individuals may be naturally short, stocky, or muscular, no one is naturally plump. The primary function of fat is storage of excess energy in times of plenty so that it is available for use when food is scarce. An abundance of permanent fat doesn't suit this purpose, but is an *unnatural* condition resulting from the overabundance of highly palatable food in the modern environment.

In order to reach a more natural body form, you must either change your environment or compensate for the overabundance of highly palatable food in some other way. The bottom line is that if you consume more energy (calories) than your body needs, you gain fat, and if you consume less, you lose it. That is the nature of fat.

"Gaining weight is a natural part of aging."

The only way to gain fat is to eat more calories than you burn. Older people tend to have more fat than younger people for the same reason they tend to have more money: they have had more time to accumulate it. Also, most of us live in a more fattening food environment and are less active than in our younger years.

Although the resting metabolic rate of most adults slows with age due to loss of muscle and organ mass,[14] this can be reversed with strengthening and endurance exercises.[15-18] Alternatively, if you don't want to go to the effort of keeping your metabolism up, you can prevent weight gain by eating fewer calories to match your slower metabolism.

"You have a natural weight that your body returns to when you are not dieting."

You do not have a single natural weight. The weight that is natural for your body depends on how many calories you eat and how physically active you are.

If you begin eating more calories each day or become less physically active, you will gain fat (and muscle to carry around the extra fat) until you have gained as much weight as your daily calories will support. That will be your new "natural weight."

Similarly, if you begin eating fewer calories, or burning more through exercise, your weight will naturally drop to a lower level.

"Being slim means being hungry."

Not with good eating habits. For example, keeping food out of sight between meals can help prevent cravings, and meals and snacks that are nutritionally balanced will keep you satisfied longer.

A balanced meal includes some protein and fat, as well as carbohydrates in the form of fiber-rich fruits, vegetables, or whole grains. The combination of protein, fat, and fiber in a balanced meal slows digestion and provides longer satisfaction after the meal ends. Foods made with processed grains or added sugars should be avoided or eaten in smaller amounts because they tend to digest quickly, so you are hungry sooner.

"If it says 'energy' or 'power,' it must be good for you."

Not if the first ingredient (or second, after water) is a sugar, such as sucrose, maltose, brown sugar, glucose, honey, or corn syrup. Sugars supply energy but little else in the way of nutrition. Just remember that energy in food is measured in calories. If you are overweight, you are already consuming too much energy.

"You can never be as slim as before you had children."

Fat gained during pregnancy can be lost like any other fat, by adjustments in eating and exercise habits. It can also be lost by breastfeeding, which uses about four or five hundred calories a day.

Abdominal muscle tone lost during pregnancy can be improved with exercise to create a more slender appearance.

"Eating healthy means not being able to have dessert."

Sweets and other unhealthy foods can be eaten occasionally, or even daily, as long as they are eaten in smaller portions. Smaller portions, when eaten slowly to savor each bite, can provide as much enjoyment as larger portions.

"For losing weight, the less fat you eat, the better."

Only up to a point. As far as your weight is concerned, the main problem with fat is that it is calorie dense. A cup of vegetable oil, for example, has more than twice the number of calories as a cup of sugar.

Fat is not all bad, however. A little fat in your meal can keep you satisfied longer by slowing carbohydrate digestion. Fat can also make food taste better. As a result, a diet that includes a moderate amount of fat can be easier to stick with, resulting in more long-term weight loss than would occur on a very low fat diet. In other words, extremely low fat diets encourage cheating or giving up.[19]

Some people mistakenly believe that fat-free or low-fat foods will not make them "fat." Excess calories from any source—fat, protein, or carbohydrate—will promote weight gain.

"Dietary supplements make losing weight much easier."

No supplement can substitute for healthy eating and a physically active lifestyle. Extra body fat is caused by extra calories, and in order to remove it, you need to eat less or burn more. You don't need a supplement for that. You just need correct information and the determination to live a healthier lifestyle.

Do some research before buying any supplement for weight loss. Words like *detoxify, purify, cleanse, miracle, ancient, secret,* and *amazing* are more often used by marketers selling overpriced products than by research scientists or medical professionals. The US Food and Drug

Administration[20] and Federal Trade Commission[21] have websites with tips and resources for evaluating claims about dietary supplements.

"How fat you are depends on the kind of bacteria in your gut."

Recent scientific studies have been interpreted this way by some.[22] What the studies really show is that certain types of bacteria in your intestines can add about 2 percent more calories to your meal by digesting components of your food that would otherwise remain undigested. This amounts to twenty to fifty calories per day for the average overweight adult. Most of us need to decrease our daily intake of calories by about ten times that amount. The effect of the bacteria is small by comparison. The studies also show that individuals who lose substantial amounts of weight lose much of the bacteria at the same time. This suggests that the abundance of the bacteria may be a result of excess fat or overeating rather than a cause.

10
Your Easiest Path
(Fifty-Six Ways to Weigh Less)

All the books in the world won't help you lose weight until you put what you have learned into practice. This chapter will help you do that. You can design your own optimized weight loss path in about five minutes, then take your first steps to being naturally thin.

As Simple as One, Two, Three
You are unique, with your own habits, abilities, and preferences, and your own reasons for your extra weight. Your easiest path to a naturally thin body is unique also. Follow the steps below to find it.

Step One
Read through the list of naturally thin habits later in the chapter. If you already have a habit, convert the circle next to it into a smiley face. Having a habit doesn't mean you are perfect at it. If you do something with 80 percent consistency, consider it a habit.

Step Two

There is a blank space after each circle. Use this space to rate the remaining habits according to how easily you could develop them. Write "1" next to the habit that would be easiest to develop, "2" next to the habit that would be the next easiest, and so on. You can find a printable version of the list at fatlossscience.org/book/path.

Step Three

Now, choose two habits that you rated as the easiest to develop, and spend a few minutes deciding exactly how you will make them your own. Turn to the chapters where the habits are discussed (see the number in parentheses after each habit) for ideas. Spend a couple of weeks focusing your efforts on these habits.

When you feel that you have mastered a habit (with 80 percent consistency), convert the circle next to it into a smiley face, and choose the next easiest one to work on.

As you travel along this path from habit "1" to habit "2" to habit "3" and so forth, you will gradually stop gaining weight and start losing it. The farther along the path you travel, the more weight you will lose as each new habit brings you closer to your naturally thin potential. You don't have to develop all of these habits, but each one will help you lose weight, and as long as you keep your new habits, the weight won't come back.

By starting with the habits that are easiest to develop, you will experience the rewards of success right away, and those early rewards will give you extra motivation to tackle habits that require more effort. After two or three weeks with a new habit, it will begin to feel natural, and you will be a naturally thinner person.

Naturally Thin Habits

◯___ Practice focusing on the present most days (Ch 3)

◯___ Practice relaxation for twelve minutes most days (Ch 3)

◯___ Practice healthy thinking most days (Ch 3)

◯___ Interact socially on a regular basis (Ch 3)

◯___ Develop a skill, create art, or help others regularly (Ch 3)

◯___ Keep your home mostly junk food free (Ch 4)

◯___ Keep your work space mostly junk food free (Ch 4)

◯___ Decide in advance what to do in tempting situations (Ch 4)

◯___ Master one method for calming cravings (Ch 4)

◯___ Master three methods for calming cravings (Ch 4)

◯___ Use a binge-prevention technique as needed (Ch 4)

◯___ Use self-therapy for cravings as needed (Ch 4)

◯___ Eat a handful of nuts with breakfast most days (Ch 6)

◯___ Eat a handful of nuts with lunch or dinner most days (Ch 6)

◯___ Eat vegetables or fresh fruit with breakfast most days (Ch 6)

◯___ Eat vegetables or fresh fruit for a third of lunch most days (Ch 6)

◯___ Eat vegetables or fresh fruit for half of lunch most days (Ch 6)

◯___ Eat vegetables or fresh fruit for a third of dinner most days (Ch 6)

○ ___ Eat vegetables or fresh fruit for half of dinner most days (Ch 6)

○ ___ Eat slowly-digesting grains with breakfast most days (Ch 6)

○ ___ Eat slowly-digesting grains with lunch most days (Ch 6)

○ ___ Eat slowly-digesting grains with dinner most days (Ch 6)

○ ___ Eat low-fat yogurt with breakfast most days (Ch 6)

○ ___ Eat low-fat yogurt with lunch or dinner most days (Ch 6)

○ ___ Eat no more than three refined-floury or sugary foods a day (Ch 6)

○ ___ Eat no more than two refined-floury or sugary foods a day (Ch 6)

○ ___ Eat refined-floury or sugary foods only in small portions (Ch 6)

○ ___ Eat potato-based foods no more than once a week (Ch 6)

○ ___ Eat potato-based foods only in small portions (Ch 6)

○ ___ Eat white rice no more than once a week (Ch 6)

○ ___ Eat white rice only in small portions (Ch 6)

○ ___ Eat high-calorie dressings and toppings sparingly (Ch 6)

○ ___ Drink no more than one sugary or alcoholic drink a day (Ch 6)

○ ___ Drink sugary drinks no more than once a week (Ch 6)

○ ___ Drink sugary or alcoholic drinks only in small amounts (Ch 6)

○ ___ Eat breakfast, lunch, and dinner every day (Ch 6)

○ ___ Eat a solid, balanced breakfast every day (Ch 6)

○ ___ Eat junk food only with meals (Ch 6)

○ ___ Eat breakfast mindfully (Ch 6)

○ ___ Eat lunch mindfully (Ch 6)

○ ___ Eat dinner mindfully (Ch 6)

○ ___ Eat snacks mindfully, if at all (Ch 6)

○ ___ Eat restaurant food no more than six times a week (Ch 6)

○ ___ Eat restaurant food no more than three times a week (Ch 6)

○ ___ When eating out, eat a small meal (Ch 6)

○ ___ Get enough sleep (Ch 6)

○ ___ Watch television no more than one hour most days (Ch 6)

○ ___ Watch television no more than thirty minutes most days (Ch 6)

○ ___ Don't watch television most days (Ch 6)

○ ___ Limit total leisure screen time to one hour most days (Ch 7)

○ ___ Exercise at least ten minutes most days (Ch 7)

○ ___ Exercise at least thirty minutes most days (Ch 7)

○ ___ Exercise at least forty-five minutes most days (Ch 7)

○ ___ Exercise at least sixty minutes most days (Ch 7)

○ ___ Do three or more strengthening exercises at least twice a week (Ch 8)

○ ___ Do six or more strengthening exercises at least twice a week (Ch 8)

If you already have some of these habits, congratulations! You are already part way down the path to naturally thin. Now keep moving forward by developing the next easiest habit.

If you lose your footing and slide back a step or two, don't give up. Consider it a learning experience, find creative solutions to your challenges, and try again. Slow, persistent improvement in your habits will bring lasting rewards.

Having a companion on your journey can help you stay on track and work through difficulties. Consider inviting your spouse or a friend to read this book and take some of these life-changing steps with you.

 QuickStart Tip*—Spend a few minutes to find at least one or two things to do right now to begin forming the next easiest habit.*

Measuring Success

Don't expect to lose weight quickly. This isn't a diet, after all. Your goal should be permanent, not rapid, weight loss. Losing even a half pound a week that doesn't come back is better than losing four pounds that do. Permanent weight loss is best accomplished by gradually losing weight based on long-term changes in habits. When you first gained the extra weight, you probably gained it gradually, one habit at a time. Let yourself lose it the same way.

Your weight loss may also be slowed a bit, in a good way, if you are gaining muscle with strengthening exercises. Muscle is heavy, but it promotes a shapely figure. If you are gaining muscle at the same time you are losing fat, you will look thinner even if you can't see a difference on the scale.

Instead of trying to track your weight loss by getting on the scale every morning, try this. Once a week, stand in front of the mirror, smile, and ask yourself, "Do I look better than I did a week ago? Do I feel healthier? Do my clothes feel a little looser?" If the answer to any of these questions is yes, you are making real progress.

The best of success on your weight loss adventure!

Appendix A
Simple Vegetable Recipes

When it comes to food, many weight loss books have it wrong. They ask you to replace the convenient foods you've eaten all your life with rigid, detailed menus or complex recipes. Who's going to keep that up for very long? Most of us don't have the time or mental energy to change our entire way of eating or prepare complex recipes.

The truth is that you don't need to give up the convenient foods you've been eating. Just eat them in smaller portions and less often. Make up the difference with low-fat yogurt, slowly-digesting grains, and unprocessed fruits, nuts, and vegetables. The addition of these weight loss foods to your meals will enable you to eat smaller portions of less-healthy foods without going hungry. As a result, you will consume fewer calories, be satisfied longer after a meal ends, and be less tempted to snack.

Adding weight loss foods to your meals will be easy with the recipes in these appendices. Most have six or fewer ingredients, take only a few minutes to prepare, and require only minimal cooking skills.

Roasted Vegetables

The high temperatures used in roasting enhance the flavor of vegetables by caramelizing the naturally occurring sugars. You can roast almost any vegetable. Asparagus, beets, bell peppers, broccoli, brussels sprouts, cauliflower, corn on the cob, carrots, eggplant, green beans, mushrooms, onions, parsnips, summer squash, sweet potatoes, turnips, and zucchini work well.

Preheat oven to 420° F. Cut an assortment of **vegetables** into 1-inch pieces. Dense vegetables such as beets, parsnips, and carrots should be cut a little thinner to allow faster cooking. Toss the cut pieces with a little **salt** and **oil** in a bowl until each piece is lightly coated. Spread in a single layer on a baking sheet. Place in oven. When the undersides of the pieces have started to brown (about 10–15 minutes), turn them over. Remove when the undersides have started to brown again (about 10 minutes more).

If the vegetables are still too firm, cut them thinner or use a lower oven temperature the next time. If they are too dry or mushy, use a higher temperature or cut them thicker. For variety, include a little basil, parsley, rosemary, thyme, pepper, or marjoram in the oil mix used for tossing.

Roasted vegetables can be eaten many different ways. Try them with plain yogurt or yogurt dip, sprinkled with vinegar, pepper, or Parmesan cheese, dressed up with fresh thyme or oregano, tossed with pasta or nuts, mixed with seasoned rice, or added to salads.

Vegetables in Fried Eggs

Try this recipe with fresh bell peppers, spinach, zucchini, tomatoes, mushrooms, asparagus, or canned nopales.

Cut **vegetables** into bite-sized pieces and fry in oil for a few minutes. Season with **salt** and **pepper**. Crack an **egg** or two over the vegetables and fry in whatever manner you prefer.

Alternatively, add leftover roasted vegetables, or some fresh avocado or tomato to your eggs after they are cooked.

Steamed Vegetables

Steamed vegetables are simple, versatile, nutritious, low-calorie, and will help make any meal more satisfying. Try the following recipe with cauliflower, green beans, cabbage, brussels sprouts, broccoli, zucchini, sweet potatoes, or carrots.

Slice **vegetables** into ½-inch pieces. Place in a pot with about an inch of **water,** or in a steamer. Cover with a lid. Bring the water to a boil and steam the vegetables until they just start to soften or become slightly translucent. This should take 4 to 10 minutes. Don't overcook, or they will become too soft and lose color and flavor. Drain. **Salt** to taste.

Eat with a little vinegar, lemon juice, or plain low-fat yogurt to take away any bitterness that may be present, or with a little olive oil for flavor.

Steamed Greens

Greens are the edible leaves of vegetables. They are high in vitamins, antioxidants, and fiber, and very low in calories. The simplest, quickest way to prepare greens is by steaming. Try the following recipe using spinach, beet greens, Swiss chard, or mustard greens. Don't worry, greens cooked this way will *not* taste like canned spinach.

Take a large handful of fresh greens or 2 cups of frozen **greens**. If you are using fresh greens, rinse them well. Place in a steamer or in a pan with an inch or two of **water**. Cover with a lid. Bring to a boil, then turn down the heat and simmer until the leaves reach the desired softness (10–20 minutes). Drain. **Salt** to taste.

Eat with a little vinegar, lemon juice, or plain low-fat yogurt to take away any bitterness that may be present, or with a little olive oil for flavor.

Makes 2 servings.

Dipped Vegetables

Fresh, crispy vegetable pieces eaten with a tasty yogurt dip can be almost as tempting as potato chips, and much better for losing weight. Try cherry tomatoes, baby carrots, snow peas, snap peas, cauliflower, broccoli, zucchini, cucumber, celery, or sweet potato.

Cut **vegetables** into bite-sized pieces. Make a dip by mixing ¼ cup of your favorite **salad dressing** with ½ cup **plain low-fat yogurt,** or use a yogurt dip recipe from appendix C.

Stir-Fried Vegetables

Prepare 4 cups of vegetables cut up into pieces less than ½-inch thick. Keep slow-cooking vegetables such as onions, carrots, asparagus, broccoli, and bell peppers separate from fast-cooking vegetables such as zucchini, yellow squash, and snow peas.

In a wok or large skillet, heat 1½ tablespoons **peanut, sesame, or canola oil** over medium-high heat. Peanut or sesame oil will provide more flavor than canola oil. Don't heat the oil so much that it smokes. Add the slow-cooking **vegetables** and stir constantly for 1 minute, then add the fast-cooking vegetables and stir for 2 minutes. Add 3 tablespoons **soy sauce or** 5 tablespoons **teriyaki sauce** and continue to stir for 2 more minutes.

Eat with pasta or brown rice.

Makes 4 servings.

Mint and Honey Carrots

Peel 4 medium **carrots** and cut into bite-sized pieces. Steam or simmer in ½ inch of **water** until tender. Drain. Add 1 teaspoon **oil or butter**, 1 teaspoon **honey**, a pinch of **salt**, and ¼ teaspoon **dried mint leaves**.

For variety, substitute parsnips, cauliflower, or turnips for the carrots.

Makes 3 to 4 servings.

Fun Green Salads

Here's a simple formula for a fun, healthy, satisfying salad:

Green base + bright color + fun flavor or texture + protein

Start with a green base of **lettuce, spinach, cabbage, sprouts, or snow peas.** Add a **brightly colored fruit or vegetable** to make the salad visually appealing. Then add an **intense flavor or crunchy, soft, or chewy texture** to make it fun to eat. Finally, add some **protein** to make it satisfying. You can create an endless variety of fun salads with just four ingredients. Here are some ideas:

- fresh spinach, sliced strawberries, chopped walnuts, feta
- lettuce, grated carrots, sliced tomatoes, hard-boiled egg
- romaine lettuce, dried cranberries, diced celery, Parmesan
- green leaf lettuce, sliced tomatoes, olives, feta
- fresh spinach, mandarin orange segments, crunchy chow mein noodles, sliced almonds
- lettuce, sliced pepperoncini, cucumber, hard-boiled egg
- fresh spinach, dried cranberries, chopped pecans, feta
- lettuce, sliced tomatoes, avocado, chopped chicken breast
- snow peas, sliced apple, mandarin orange sections, peanuts
- lettuce, purple grapes, feta, chickpeas
- lettuce, diced red bell pepper, green grapes, feta

Eat with a little light dressing. See appendix C for recipes.

Instant Tomato Soup

Pour **tomato or vegetable juice,** such as V8®, into a pan. Bring to a low boil.

Eat topped with whole-grain crackers, a spoonful of yogurt, or a little feta, Parmesan, or grated cheddar.

Garden Vegetable Soup

Try this recipe using any of the following vegetables: onions, celery, sweet potatoes, carrots, tomatoes, zucchini, yellow squash, green beans, corn, or shredded cabbage. Dense, slow-cooking vegetables such as carrots and sweet potatoes should be cut into ¼-inch thick pieces. Most others can be cut into ½-inch thick pieces.

Combine 4 cups of **vegetables** with 6 cups of **chicken or vegetable stock.** You can buy stock in cans or reconstitute it from base or bullion. Bring the soup to a boil and then simmer until vegetables are tender (20–30 minutes). **Salt** to taste.

For variety, add 1 teaspoon parsley, ½ teaspoon basil, or a pinch of thyme to the simmering soup.

Makes about 6 servings.

Baked Winter Squash

Winter squash are hard-skinned varieties of squash such as butternut, delicata, acorn, and banana squash.

Cut **squash** in half lengthwise. Remove the seeds and scrape away any stringy layer with a spoon. Place the two halves cut-side up in a baking dish. Add ¼ inch of **water** to the baking dish to keep the squash from drying out. Dab the cut surface with **oil or warm butter** and sprinkle with **brown sugar** and a little **salt**. Bake at 400° until the flesh is soft (about 40–70 minutes).

For variety, try cinnamon, cumin, coriander, mustard, or honey instead of brown sugar.

Eat as a side dish, plain or topped with yogurt.

Appendix B
Simple Whole Grain Recipes

The recipes in these appendices are for basic foods, much like our ancestors might have eaten before the current weight gain epidemic. They have simple flavors that you won't soon tire of. They taste good enough to be satisfying, but not so good that you can't stop eating them. Learn to appreciate their natural flavors and textures.

If you don't want to use sugar or one of the other sweeteners used in these recipes, try substituting a different sweetener. Just be aware of the calories you are adding. Calories from any sweetener, no matter how "natural" it is, will contribute to weight gain.

Seasoned Brown Basmati Rice

If you don't like the brown rice you have tasted in the past, you are not alone. Give brown *basmati* rice a chance. Basmati is known for a pleasant flavor. It really doesn't need any seasoning, just a little salt, but you can add seasonings for variety. If you can't find brown basmati rice in your local grocery store, try a health food store or the Internet.

Place 2 cups **brown basmati rice,** 3¼ cups **water,** 1 tablespoon **oil,** and ¼ teaspoon **salt** in a pan. Add ½ teaspoon dried **dill weed, mint, or parsley.** Cover with a lid. Bring to a boil, then turn the heat down and simmer until the water is gone. Turn the heat off and let the rice sit for 15 minutes before eating. You may need to slightly adjust the amount of water to achieve the proper texture, which should be al dente.

For variety, substitute converted rice for the brown rice, or add a little wild rice. Substitute 2 teaspoons lemon juice for the herb.

Eat with lunch or dinner as a side dish or topped with vegetables.

Makes 6 to 8 servings.

Brown Basmati Rice for Breakfast

Brown basmati rice makes an excellent hot breakfast cereal that will keep you satisfied for hours.

Follow the recipe for **Seasoned Brown Basmati Rice,** but instead of adding any of the herbs mentioned in the recipe, try chopped **dried fruit or** ¼ teaspoon **ground nutmeg, ground cinnamon, or anise seed.**

Eat the rice as a hot cereal in milk and topped with fruit, nuts, or a little honey.

Makes 6 to 8 servings.

Oatmeal

Avoid single-serving packages of instant oatmeal, which may contain about as much sugar as they do oats. Instead, try regular (old-fashioned) rolled oats or steel-cut oats. While oatmeal cooked using regular rolled oats is creamy, oatmeal from steel-cut oats is firmer.

Boil 2 cups of **water**. Add a pinch of **salt** and 1 cup **regular rolled oats or steel-cut oats**. Stir once and remove from heat. Let it sit covered for 10 minutes. If the oatmeal comes out thicker than you like it, use more water. You can substitute milk for some or all of the water for a richer flavor. If you want the oatmeal creamier, stir it for a minute before removing from the heat.

Eat with milk and fresh fruit, raisins or other dried fruit, nuts, or a little honey.

Makes 2 to 4 servings.

Fried Oatmeal

Place 2 cups **leftover cooked oatmeal** in a plastic container and press it down to remove the air spaces. Leave it in the refrigerator overnight to cool and solidify. Remove the oatmeal from the container in one piece and cut it into ¼-inch thick slices. Fry the slices in a small amount of **oil** over medium heat. When the slices have browned on the bottom, flip them over to brown on the other side.

Eat dribbled with a little molasses or jam.

Makes 2 to 4 servings.

Hulled Millet

Place 2 cups **hulled millet,** 3½ cups **water,** 1 tablespoon oil, and ¼ teaspoon **salt** in a pan. Let it sit 1 hour. Cover with a lid and bring to a boil. Turn the heat down and simmer until the water is gone, then remove from heat and let it sit 15 minutes.

Eat as a substitute for rice, or as a hot cereal with milk and topped with fruit or nuts. You can also add a little honey to make it more satisfying.

Makes 6 to 8 servings.

Bulgur

Bulgur is wheat that has been steamed or boiled, dried, and then crushed.

Place 2 cups **medium-ground bulgur,** 3½ cups **water,** 1 tablespoon **oil,** and ¼ teaspoon **salt** in a pan. Cover with a lid and bring to a boil. Turn the heat down and simmer until the water is gone, then remove from heat and let it sit 15 minutes.

Use the bulgur like rice, or as a hot breakfast cereal in milk and topped with fruit, nuts, or a little jam or honey.

Makes 6 to 8 servings.

Light and Crunchy Granola

Preheat oven to 300°F. Combine ¼ cup **plain low-fat yogurt**, ¼ cup **brown sugar**, 1 teaspoon **ground cinnamon**, and ¼ teaspoon **salt**. Mix well. Add 2 cups **rolled oats** and ½ cup **chopped nuts or seeds**. Pecans, cashews, walnuts, slivered almonds, peanuts, sunflower seeds, sesame seeds, and pumpkin seeds all work well. Stir until all of the rolled oats are moistened. Spread the mixture ½ inch deep on a cookie sheet. Bake until some of the granola begins to brown (about 20–30 minutes). Allow to cool before eating.

Most granola recipes call for oil or syrup instead of yogurt. Yogurt gives the granola a lighter taste and fewer calories.

For variety, add some shredded coconut to the mix, or use different nuts. To make a lighter granola, substitute puffed wheat for some of the rolled oats.

Enjoy the granola in low-fat milk or yogurt, topped with raisins or fresh fruit.

Makes 6 to 8 servings.

Appendix C
Simple Yogurt Recipes

Try the Easy Homemade Yogurt recipe on the following page to make your own inexpensive, additive-free, low-calorie yogurt. You can then use it or any plain low-fat yogurt in the other recipes.

Plain yogurt is a very versatile food. It can be eaten with almost any meal as a side dish or as a topping in place of sour cream, sauce, or dressing. Try it as a topping on desserts to balance the sweetness. If you don't like plain yogurt at first, give it some time. It may take a while to get used to.

If you prefer flavored yogurt, add just a little jelly, jam, or honey to plain yogurt.

Easy Homemade Yogurt

This recipe has five short steps:

1. Stir ¾ cup **non-fat dry milk** into 2 quarts **1 percent milk**.

2. Heat it to 180°F.

3. Let it cool to 120°F.

4. Stir ¼ cup **plain low-fat yogurt** into the milk as a starter.

5. Keep the milk warm for at least 3 hours.

It's probably easiest to heat the milk in a double boiler or in a glass bowl in a microwave. If you prefer, you can heat the milk in a heavy pan over medium heat, but you will need to stir it to keep it from sticking to the bottom of the pan.

Any brand of plain yogurt should work for the starter as long as it has "live, active cultures" in the list of ingredients. Use a container of yogurt that hasn't been previously opened, and check its expiration date. Also, make sure that anything that touches the cooled milk or starter is clean so as not to introduce foreign bacteria or enzymes that might interfere with the yogurt-making process.

To keep the milk warm (step five), put it in a container with a lid and place it in a picnic cooler. Add hot tap water (110–120°) to the cooler to surround the milk and help keep it warm. To become yogurt, the milk must stay above 100° for about 3 hours. The longer it's kept warm, the tangier and firmer the yogurt will be.

When the yogurt is done, you may see whey, a yellowish liquid, separating out. That's normal for yogurt that doesn't have added stabilizers.

Save ¼ cup of the newly made yogurt to use as a starter for the next batch. For best results, use the starter within a couple of weeks. If you don't like the texture of your first batch of yogurt, try it again using a different brand of yogurt as a starter.

Makes about 12 servings.

Greek Yogurt

Greek yogurt is a thick, creamy yogurt made by straining regular yogurt to remove some of the liquid.

Line a strainer or colander with cheesecloth or a coffee filter. Add **plain low-fat yogurt** (without added stabilizers). Let the liquid drain off for at least two hours.

Use Greek yogurt for making spreads, topping or dips, or in recipes as a low-calorie substitute for sour cream or cream cheese.

Tzatziki (Cucumber Yogurt Sauce)

Peel a medium **cucumber** and cut it in half lengthwise. Remove the seeds by scraping out the center portion of the cucumber with a spoon. Grate the cucumber and press it with a paper towel to remove the extra liquid. Mix the grated cucumber with 2 cups **Greek yogurt**, 1 tablespoon fresh **dill or mint** (or 1 teaspoon dried dill weed or mint), 1 tablespoon **vinegar or lemon juice**, 1 tablespoon **olive oil** (optional), and ¼ teaspoon **salt**. Chill for 2 hours before serving. Add a crushed clove of **garlic** if desired.

Eat with any hot dish or use as a spread or vegetable dip. To make a salad dressing, use regular yogurt instead of Greek yogurt.

Low-Fat Yogurt Dip or Sauce

You can make a yogurt sauce or dip with almost any herb, spice, or chopped dried fruit as a flavoring. Try dill weed, mint, parsley, chives, scallion, cumin, curry powder, dried apricots, or dried cranberries.

To a bowl, add 2 cups of **regular or Greek yogurt.** The Greek yogurt will make a thicker sauce or dip. Add your preferred **flavoring** (use 1 tablespoon of a fresh herb, a teaspoon of a dried herb, ½ teaspoon of a spice, or ¼ cup of finely chopped dried fruit). Add 1 tablespoon **vinegar**. Add **salt or pepper** to taste. Mix well.

Eat with any hot dish, as a spread on crackers, or as a dip for fresh vegetables.

Low-Fat Yogurt Salad Dressing

Follow the recipe for **Low-Fat Yogurt Dip or Sauce** using regular instead of Greek yogurt. Add 1 tablespoon **vinegar** and 3 tablespoons **olive oil**. If it is still too thick, add more oil or vinegar.

Makes about 20 servings.

Quick Light Salad Dressing

For a light dressing, take ¼ cup of any **salad dressing** and mix it with ½ cup **plain low-fat yogurt**.

Makes about 6 servings.

Yogurt Parfait

To a cup of **plain low-fat yogur**t, add a few drops of vanilla and a little **sugar or honey** if desired. Mix well. Top or layer with **fruit, chopped or sliced nuts, grated coconut, granola, or whole grain breakfast cereal.**

Eat for breakfast, as a snack, or as a dessert.

Makes 1 or 2 servings.

Yogurt Fruit Dip or Fruit Salad

Combine 1 cup **plain low-fat regular or Greek yogurt** with 1 tablespoon **brown sugar, honey, or jam**. Mix well. Chill for 30 minutes.

For variety, add 1 tablespoon lemon juice or ½ teaspoon ground cinnamon or vanilla.

Eat with bite-sized pieces of apples, strawberries, grapes, or other fruit, or mix it with chopped fruit to make a fruit salad.

Makes about 6 servings.

Mango Lassi (Mango Yogurt Drink)

In a blender, combine 2½ cups **plain low-fat yogurt**, ¾ cup frozen peeled **mango**, and ¼ cup **sugar**. Blend until smooth.

To take full advantage of mango lassi's weight loss potential, take small sips and savor each one. Whether you drink it as a snack or in a meal, taking several minutes to enjoy this drink will give your stomach time to register satisfaction, and will make eating anything else seem boring in comparison.

Makes 3 servings.

Yogurt Chicken Stroganoff

Add 1 tablespoon **oil**, ½ cup chopped **onion**, 1 cup chopped **skinless chicken breast or ground turkey**, ¼ cup chopped **mushrooms,** ¼ teaspoon **salt**, and a little **pepper** to a skillet. Add a pinch of **dill weed, parsley, or garlic**. Stir over medium heat until the meat is cooked. Stir 1 tablespoon cornstarch into ½ cup cold water and add it to the mixture in the skillet. Stir until thickened, then remove from the heat. Stir in 1 cup **plain low-fat yogurt** just before eating over pasta, brown basmati rice, bulgur, or hulled millet.

Makes 6 servings.

References

Chapter 1—Why the Weight?

1. National Institutes of Health. 2010. "Overweight and obesity statistics." *Weight-Control Information Network*. http://win .niddk.nih.gov/statistics/index.htm.

2. Peters, J.C. 2002. "The challenge of managing body weight in the modern world." *Asia Pacific Journal of Clinical Nutrition* 11:S714–S717.

3. French, S.A., M. Story, and R.W. Jeffery. 2001. "Environmental influences on eating and physical activity." *Annual Review of Public Health* 22:309–335.

4. Centers for Disease Control and Prevention. 2004. "Trends in intake of energy and macronutrients—United States, 1971–2000." *Morbidity and Mortality Weekly Report* 53:80–82.

5. Wright, J.D. and C.Y. Wang. 2010. "Trends in intake of energy and macronutrients in adults from 1999–2000 through 2007–2008." *NCHS Data Brief* 51:1–8.

6. Bottom Line Health. 2009. "Your taste buds are being fooled!" *Bottom Line Health*. http://www.bottomlinepublications.com/ content/drafts/your-taste-buds-are-being-fooled.

7. Johnson, P.M. and P.J. Kenny. 2010. "Dopamine D2 receptors in addiction-like reward dysfunction and compulsive eating in obese rats." *Nature Neuroscience* 13:635–641.

8. Prentice, A. and S. Jebb. 2004. "Energy intake/physical activity interactions in the homeostasis of body weight regulation." *Nutrition Reviews* 62:S98–S104.

9. Levine, A.S. and C.J. Billington. 2004. "Why do we eat? A neural systems approach." *Annual Review of Nutrition* 17:597–619.

10. Wansink, B. 2004. "Environmental factors that increase the food intake and consumption volume of unknowing consumers." *Annual Review of Nutrition* 24:455–479.

11. Young, L.R. and M. Nestle. 2002. "The contribution of expanding portion sizes in the US obesity epidemic." *American Journal of Public Health* 92:246–249.

12. Briefel, R. and C. Johnson. 2004. "Secular trends in dietary intake in the United States." *Annual Review of Nutrition* 24:401–431.

13. Aldana, S. 2005. *The Culprit and the Cure: Why Lifestyle is the Culprit behind America's Poor Health.* Mapleton, Utah: Maple Mountain Press.

Chapter 2—Why Diets Fail

1. Centers for Disease Control and Prevention. June 2010. *Healthy Weight—It's Not a Diet, It's a Lifestyle!* http://www.cdc.gov/healthyweight/index.html.

2. Thomas, S.L., J. Hyde, A. Karunaratne, R. Kausman and P.A. Komesaroff. 2008. "'They all work…when you stick to them': A qualitative investigation of dieting, weight loss, and physical exercise, in obese individuals." *Nutrition Journal* 7:34.

3. Mann, T., A.J. Tomiyama, E. Westling, A.M. Lew, B. Samuels, and J. Chatman. 2007. "Medicare's search for effective obesity

treatments: diets are not the answer." *American Psychologist* 62:220–33.

4. US Department of Agriculture and US Department of Health and Human Services. 2010. *Dietary Guidelines for Americans, 2010.* Washington, DC: US Government Printing Office.

Chapter 3—Emotional Eating

1. Berridge, K.C., C.Y. Ho, J.M. Richard, and A.G. DiFeliceantonio. 2010. "The tempted brain eats: pleasure and desire circuits in obesity and eating." *Brain Research* 1350:43–64.

2. Berridge, K.C.,T.E. Robinson, and J.W. Aldridge. 2009. "Dissecting components of reward: 'liking', 'wanting', and learning." *Current Opinion in Pharmacology* 9:65–73.

3. Avena, N.M., P. Rada, and B.G. Hoebel. 2008. "Evidence for sugar addiction: behavioral and neurochemical effects of intermittent, excessive sugar intake." *Neuroscience and Biobehavioral Review* 32:20–39.

4. Johnson, P.M. and P.J. Kenny. 2010. "Dopamine D2 receptors in addiction-like reward dysfunction and compulsive eating in obese rats." *Nature Neuroscience* 13:635–641.

5. Killingsworth, M.A. and D.T. Gilbert. 2010. "A wandering mind is an unhappy mind." *Science* 330:932.

6. Baer, R.A. 2003. "Mindfulness training as a clinical intervention: a conceptual and empirical review." *Clinical Psychology: Science and Practice* 10:125–143.

7. Majzoub, J.A. 2006. "Corticotropin-releasing hormone physiology." *European Journal of Endocrinology* 155:S71–S76.

8. Esch, T., G.L. Fricchione, and G.B. Stefano. 2003. "The therapeutic use of the relaxation response in stress-related diseases." *Medical Sciences Monitor* 9:RA23–34.

9. Benson, H., and W. Proctor. 2010. *Relaxation Revolution: Enhancing Your Personal Health through the Science and Genetics of Mind Body Healing.* New York, NY: Scribner.

10. Chiesa, A. and A. Serretti. 2010. "A systematic review of neurobiological and clinical features of mindfulness meditations." *Psychological Medicine* 40:1239–1252.

11. Holzel, B.K., J. Carmody, K.C. Evans, E.A. Hoge, J.A. Dusek, L. Morgan, R.K. Pitman, and S.W. Lazar. 2010. "Stress reduction correlates with structural changes in the amygdala." *Social Cognitive and Affective Neuroscience* 5:11–17.

12. Strohle, A. 2009. "Physical activity, exercise, depression, and anxiety disorders." *Journal of Neural Transmission* 116:777–784.

13. Salmon, P. 2001. "Effects of physical exercise on anxiety, depression, and sensitivity to stress: a unifying theory." *Clinical Psychology Review* 21:33–61.

14. Peluso, M.A. and L.H. Guerra de Andrade. 2005. "Physical activity and mental health: the association between exercise and mood." *Clinics* 60:61–70.

Chapter 4—Beat Temptation

1. Burton, P. and H. Lightowler. 2006. "An exploration of associations between food cravings and restrained, external, and emotional eating." *Appetite* 47:260.

2. Sobik, L., K. Hutchison, and L. Craighead. 2005. "Cue-elicited craving for food: a fresh approach to the study of binge eating." *Appetite* 44:253–261.

3. Hill, J. 2007. "The psychology of food craving." *Proceedings of the Nutrition Society* 66:277–285.

4. Kemps, E., M. Tiggemann, and M. Grigg. 2008. "Food cravings consume limited cognitive resources." *Journal of Experimental Psychology: Applied* 14:247–254.

5. Morewedge, C.K., Y.E. Huh, and J. Vosgerau. 2010. "Thought for food: imagined consumption reduces actual consumption." *Science* 330:1530–1533.

6. Bleich, S.N., B.J. Herring, D.D. Flagg, and T.L. Gary-Webb. 2012. "Reduction in purchases of sugar-sweetened beverages among low-income black adolescents after exposure to caloric information." *American Journal of Public Health* 0:0,e1–e7 (Posted online 15 Dec 2011).

7. Oh, H. and A.H. Taylor. 2011. "Brisk walking reduces ad libitum snacking in regular chocolate eaters during a workplace simulation." *Appetite* 58:387–392.

8. Taylor, A.H. and A.J. Oliver. 2009. "Acute effects of brisk walking on urges to eat chocolate, affect, and responses to a stressor and chocolate cue. An experimental study." *Appetite* 52:155–160.

9. Roemer, L. and S.M. Orsillo. 2002. "Expanding our conceptualization of and treatment for generalized anxiety disorder: integrating mindfulness/acceptance-based approaches with existing cognitive-behavioral models." *Clinical Psychology: Science & Practice* 9:54–68.

10. Bishop, S.R., M. Lau, S. Shapiro, L. Carlson, N.D. Anderson, J. Carmody, Z.V. Segal, S. Abbey, M. Speca, D. Velting, and G. Devins. 2004. "Mindfulness: a proposed operational definition." *Clinical Psychology: Science & Practice* 11:230–241.

11. Baer, R.A. 2003. "Mindfulness training as a clinical intervention: a conceptual and empirical review." *Clinical Psychology: Science and Practice* 10:125–143.

12. Forman, E.M., K.L. Hoffman, K.B. McGrath, J.D. Herbert, L.L. Brandsma, and M.R. Lowe. 2007. "A comparison of acceptance- and control-based strategies for coping with food cravings: an analog study." *Behaviour Research and Therapy* 45:2372–2386.

Chapter 5—How It Adds Up

1. Centers for Disease Control and Prevention. *Overweight and Obesity: Causes and Consequences.* Centers for Disease Control and Prevention. http://www.cdc.gov/obesity/causes/index.html.

2. Manore, M., N.L. Meyer, and J. Thompson. 2009. *Sport Nutrition for Health and Performance. Second edition.* Champaign, IL: Human Kinetics.

3. Westcott, W.L. 2005. "Why every senior should do strength exercise." *Wellness.MA.* http://wellness.ma/senior-fitness/senior-fitness.htm.

4. Poehlman, E.T. 1989. "A review: exercise and its influence on resting energy metabolism in man." *Medicine and Science in Sports and Exercise* 21:515–525.

Chapter 6—Eat Less

1. Mozaffarian, D., T. Hao, E.B. Rimm, W.C. Willett, and F.B. Hu. 2011. "Changes in diet and lifestyle and long-term weight gain in women and men." *New England Journal of Medicine* 364:2392–2404.

2. Anderson, G.H. and D. Woodend. 2003. "Effect of glycemic carbohydrates on short-term satiety and food intake." *Nutrition Reviews* 61:17–26.

3. Ferrazzano, G.F., T. Cantile, M. Quarto, A. Ingenito, L. Chianese, and F. Addeo. 2008. "Protective effect of yogurt extract on dental enamel demineralization in vitro." *Australian Dental Journal* 53:314–319.

4. US Department of Agriculture and US Department of Health and Human Services. 2010. *Dietary Guidelines for Americans, 2010.* Washington, DC: US Government Printing Office.

5. Durtschi, A. 2001. *Nutritional Content of Whole Grains versus Their Refined Flours.* Washington, DC: US Department of Agriculture Economic Research Service, Walton Feed.

6. Harvard School of Public Health. "Health gains from whole grains." *The Nutrition Source.* http://www.hsph.harvard.edu/nutritionsource/what-should-you-eat/health-gains-from-whole-grains/index.html.

7. Heaton, K.W., S.N. Marcus, P.M. Emmett, and C.H. Bolton. 1988. "Particle size of wheat, maize, and oat test meals: effects on plasma glucose and insulin responses and on the rate of starch digestion in vitro." *American Journal of Clinical Nutrition* 47:675–682.

8. Jenkins, D.J., V. Wesson, T.M. Wolever, A.L. Jenkins, J. Kalmusky, S. Guidici, A. Csima, R.G. Josse, and G.S. Wong. 1988. "Wholemeal versus wholegrain breads: proportion of whole or cracked grain and the glycaemic response." *British Medical Journal* 297:958–960.

9. Juntunen, K.S., D.E. Laaksonen, K. Autio, L.K. Niskanen, J.J. Holst, K.E. Savolainen, K-H. Liukkonen, K.S. Poutanen, and H.M. Mykkänen. 2003. "Structural differences between rye and wheat breads but not total fiber content may explain the lower postprandial insulin response to rye bread." *American Journal of Clinical Nutrition* 78:957-964.

10. Anderson, G.H., C.E. Cho, T. Akhavan, R.C. Mollard, B.L. Luhovyy, and E.T. Finocchiaro. 2010. "Relation between estimates of cornstarch digestibility by the Englyst in vitro method and glycemic response, subjective appetite, and short-term food intake in young men." *American Journal of Clinical Nutrition* 91:932–939.

11. Stubbs, J., S. Ferres, and G. Horgan. 2000. "Energy density of foods: effects on energy intake." *Critical Reviews in Food Science and Nutrition* 40:481–515.

12. Jakubowicz, D., D. Maman, and P. Essah. 2008. "Effect of diet with high carbohydrate and protein breakfast on weight loss and appetite in obese women with metabolic syndrome." *ENDO meeting 2008*: Abstract P3–220.

13. Gross, L.S., L. Li, E.S. Ford, and S. Liu. 2004. "Increased consumption of refined carbohydrates and the epidemic of type 2 diabetes in the United States: an ecologic assessment." *American Journal of Clinical Nutrition* 79:774–779.

14. Geier, A.B., P. Rozin, and G. Doros. 2006. "Unit bias: a new heuristic that helps explain the effect of portion size on food intake." *Psychological Science* 17:521–525.

15. US Department of Health and Human Services. 2003. *Portion Distortion I.* http://hp2010.nhlbihin.net/portion.

16. Gangwisch, J.E., D. Malaspina, B. Boden-Albala, and S.B. Heymsfield. 2005. "Inadequate sleep as a risk factor for obesity: analyses of the NHANES I." *Sleep* 28:1289–1296.

17. Raynor, D.A., S. Phelan, J.O. Hill, and R.R. Wing. 2006. "Television viewing and long-term weight maintenance: results from the National Weight Control Registry." *Obesity* 14:1816–1824.

18. Kubey, R. and M. Csikszentmihalyi. 2002. "Television addiction is no mere metaphor." *Scientific American* 286:74–80.

Chapter 7—Be Active

1. US Department of Health and Human Services. 2008. *2008 Physical Activity Guidelines for Americans.* Washington, DC: US Government Printing Office.

2. Catenacci, V.A., L.G. Ogden, J. Stuht, S. Phelan, R.R. Wing, J.O. Hill, and H.R. Wyatt. 2008. "Physical activity patterns in the National Weight Control Registry." *Obesity* 16:153–161.

Chapter 8—Boost Your Metabolism

1. Van Pelt, R.E., F.A. Dinneno, D.R. Seals, and P.P. Jones. 2001. "Age-related decline in RMR in physically active men: relation to exercise volume and energy intake." *American Journal of Physiology—Endocrinology and Metabolism* 281:E633–E639.

2. Van Pelt, R.E., P.P. Jones, K.P. Davy, C.A. DeSouza, H. Tanaka, B.M. Davy, and D.R. Seals. 1997. "Regular exercise and the age-related decline in resting metabolic rate in women." *Journal of Clinical Endocrinology & Metabolism* 82:3208–3212.

3. Bosy-Westphal, A., C. Eichhorn, D. Kutzner, K. Illner, M. Heller, and M.J. Müller. 2003. "The age-related decline in resting energy expenditure in humans is due to the loss of fat-free mass and to alterations in its metabolically active components." *Journal of Nutrition* 133:2356–2362.

4. Ballor, D. and E. Poehlman. 1994. "Exercise training enhances fat-free mass preservation during diet-induced weight loss: a meta analytic finding." *International Journal of Obesity* 18:35–40.

5. Westcott, W.L. 2000. "Strength training for women." *Healthy.net.* http://www.healthy.net/scr/article.asp?ID=322.

6. Westcott, W.L. 2005. "Why every senior should do strength exercise." *Wellness.MA.* http://www.wellness.ma/senior-fitness/senior-fitness.htm.

7. Westcott W.L. and J. Guy. 2005. "As young as you feel." *Wellness.MA.* http://www.wellness.ma/seniorfitness/senior-strength-training.htm.

8. Westcott, W.L. 2001. "Making bodyweight exercises more challenging." *Healthy.net.* http://www.healthy.net/scr/column.asp?lk=P12&Id=372.

9. Westcott, W.L. "Strength training: how many days per week?" *Wellness.MA.* http://healthy.net/scr/article.asp?lk=P12&Id=519.

10. Westcott, W.L. "How many repetitions?" *Wellness.MA.* http://www.healthy.net/scr/article.asp?ID=334.

11. Westcott, W.L. "Strength training for time-pressured people." *Wellness.MA.* http://www.healthy.net/scr/article.asp?ID=331.

12. Westcott, W.L. "Best of both worlds: stretching and strengthening." *Wellness.MA.* http://www.healthy.net/scr/column.asp?lk=P12&Id=239.

Chapter 9—Myths

1. Weinsier, R.L, G.R. Hunter, P.A. Zuckerman, B.E. Darnell. 2003. "Low resting and sleeping energy expenditure and fat use do not contribute to obesity in women." *Obesity Research* 11:937–944.

2. Stensel, D.J., F.P. Lin, and A.M. Nevill. 2001. "Resting metabolic rate in obese and nonobese Chinese Singaporean boys aged 13–15 y." *American Journal of Clinical Nutrition* 74:369–373.

3. Stunkard, A.J., R.I. Berkowitz, D. Schoeller, G. Maislin, and V.A. Stallings. 2004. "Predictors of body size in the first 2 y of life: a high-risk study of human obesity." *International Journal of Obesity* 28:503–513.

4. Bandini, L.G., A. Must, S.M. Phillips, E.N. Naumova, and W.H. Dietz. 2004. "Relation of body mass index and body fatness to energy expenditure: longitudinal changes from preadolescence through adolescence." *American Journal of Clinical Nutrition* 80:1262–1269.

5. Hise, M.E., D.K. Sullivan, D.J. Jacobsen, S.L. Johnson, and J.E. Donnelly. 2002. "Validation of energy intake measurements determined from observer-recorded food records and recall methods compared with the doubly labeled water method

in overweight and obese individuals." *American Journal of Clinical Nutrition* 75:263–267.

6. Cook, A., J. Pryer, and P. Shetty. 2000. "The problem of accuracy in dietary surveys. Analysis of the over 65 UK National Diet and Nutrition Survey." *Journal of Epidemiology and Community Health* 54:611–616.

7. Lichtman, S.W., K. Pisarska, E.R. Berman, M. Pestone, H. Dowling, E. Offenbacher, H. Weisel, S. Heshka, D.E. Matthews, and S.B. Heymsfield. 1992. "Discrepancy between self-reported and actual caloric intake and exercise in obese subjects." *New England Journal of Medicine* 327:1893–1898.

8. Prentice, A. and S. Jebb. 2004. "Energy intake/physical activity interactions in the homeostasis of body weight regulation." *Nutrition Reviews* 62:S98–S104.

9. Peters, J.C., H.R. Wyatt, W.T. Donahoo, and J.O. Hill. 2002. "From instinct to intellect: the challenge of maintaining healthy weight in the modern world." *Obesity Reviews* 3:69–74.

10. Fox, C.S., J. Esparza, M. Nicolson, P.H. Bennett, L.O. Schulz, M.E. Valencia, and E. Ravussin. 1998. "Is a low leptin concentration, a low resting metabolic rate, or both the expression of the 'thrifty genotype'? Results from Mexican Pima Indians." *American Journal of Clinical Nutrition* 68:1053–1057.

11. Bell, C.G., A.J. Walley, and P. Froguel. 2005. "The genetics of human obesity." *Nature Reviews Genetics* 6:221–234.

12. Weinsier. R.L. 1999. "Genes and obesity: is there reason to change our behaviors?" *Annals of Internal Medicine* 130:938–939.

13. Lowe. M.R. 2003. "Self-regulation of energy intake in the prevention and treatment of obesity: is it feasible?" *Obesity Research* 11:44S–59S.

14. Bosy-Westphal, A., C. Eichhorn, D. Kutzner, K. Illner, M. Heller, and M.J. Muller. 2003. "The age-related decline in resting energy expenditure in humans is due to the loss of fat-free mass and to alterations in its metabolically active components." *Journal of Nutrition* 133:2356–2362.

15. Westcott, W.L. and J. Guy. 2005. "As Young as You Feel." *Wellness.MA.* http://www.wellness.ma/senior-fitness/senior-strength-training.htm.

16. Westcott, W.L. 2005. "Why every senior should do strength exercise." *Wellness.MA.* http://www.wellness.ma/senior-fitness/senior-fitness.htm.

17. Van Pelt, R.E., F.A. Dinneno, D.R. Seals, and P.P. Jones. 2001. "Age-related decline in RMR in physically active men: relation to exercise volume and energy intake." *American Journal of Physiology—Endocrinology and Metabolism* 281:E633–E639.

18. Van Pelt, R.E., P.P. Jones, K.P. Davy, C.A. DeSouza, H. Tanaka, B.M. Davy, and D.R. Seals. 1997. "Regular exercise and the age-related decline in resting metabolic rate in women." *Journal of Clinical Endocrinology & Metabolism* 82:3208–3212.

19. McManus, K., L. Antinoro, and F. Sacks. 2001. "A randomized controlled trial of a moderate-fat, low-energy diet compared with a low fat, low-energy diet for weight loss in overweight adults." *International Journal of Obesity* 25:1503–1511.

20. US Department of Health and Human Services. January 2002. "Tips for the savvy supplement user: making informed

decisions and evaluating information." *US Food and Drug Administration.* http://www.fda.gov/Food/DietarySupplements/ConsumerInformation/ucm110567.htm.

21. Federal Trade Commission. 2004. "Weighing the evidence in diet ads." *Federal Trade Commission.*

22. Turnbaugh, P.J., R.E. Ley, M.A. Mahowald, V. Magrini, E.R. Mardis, and J.I. Gordon. 2006. "An obesity-associated gut microbiome with increased capacity for energy harvest." *Nature* 444:1027-1031.

Index

acceptance, 19–20
advertising
    cravings and, 31
    misleading 4
aging, weight gain and, 80
alcoholic beverages, 4, 55, 59
amylose, in rice, 51, 57

bacteria, intestinal, 83
Baked Winter Squash recipe, 100
balanced meals, 53–5, 81
basic meditation, 12, 14–16
breakfast, healthy, 53–4, 56
brisk walking, controlling cravings
    with, 35–6
Brown Basmati Rice for Breakfast
    recipe, 102
Bulgur recipe, 104

calories
    burned during exercise,
        32–3, 44
    consumed vs. burned, 41–2
    foods rich in, 2–3, 58
    metabolism and, 42–4
    reducing intake of, 45–66
    stored as fat, 41–2
carbohydrates, in balanced meals,
    53–4

catastrophizing, 18
condemning and blaming, 18
cravings, handling, 28–39
curiosity, temptations and, 33–4

desserts, healthy eating and, 82
diets
    ineffectiveness of, 7–8
    low-fat, 82
Dipped Vegetables recipe, 96
dressings and toppings
    high-calorie, 58
    recipes for, 110

Easy Homemade Yogurt recipe,
    108–9
emotional eating, causes of, 9–10
    methods for controlling, 10–23
emotional independence, 18, 20
emotions, negative, 17–21
"energy" drinks, foods, 81
entertainment, passive, 4
exercise calculators, online, 33
exercise
    calories burned during, 32–3,
        44
    controlling cravings and,
        35–6
    endurance, 71

About the Author

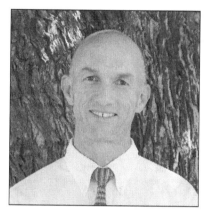

Stan Spencer, PhD, is a biological consultant with a background in research science. He has conducted laboratory studies in biochemistry at Brigham Young University, in botany and evolution at Claremont Graduate University, and in genetics at the Smithsonian Institution.

Stan lives in Southern California with his wife, Amy, and a varying number of their seven children. He enjoys hiking, birdwatching, strength training, barefoot running, and playing catch with the kids.

Stan would love to hear from you. You can drop him a note at DrStanSpencer@gmail.com or facebook.com/weightlossbook and tell him about your progress or setbacks, or give feedback on the book. Visit his blog at fatlossscience.org.

Do you have friends who could be helped by this book? Here are some ways to share it with them:

- Suggest they visit fatlossscience.org/book.
- Re-pin the book's cover from pinterest.com/weightlosstips to one of your own Pinterest boards.
- Go to fatlossscience.org/book and use one of the buttons to share the book with Facebook, Twitter, or other social media.
- "Like" the book at facebook.com/weightlossbook.
- Recommend the book at goodreads.com/stanspencer.
- Send them a link to your online review of the book.
- Use one of the sharing cards on the next page. You can find a printable version of the cards at fatlossscience.org/book.

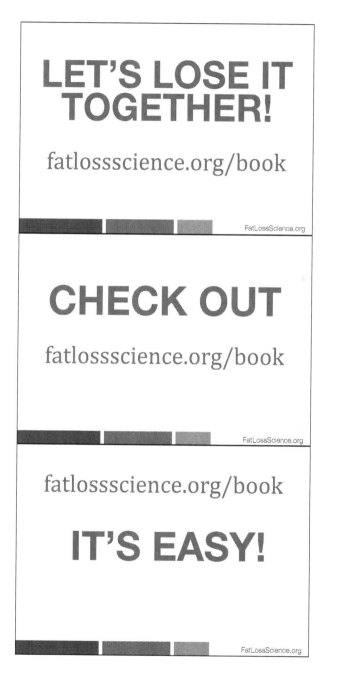

LET'S LOSE IT TOGETHER!

fatlossscience.org/book

FatLossScience.org

CHECK OUT

fatlossscience.org/book

FatLossScience.org

fatlossscience.org/book

IT'S EASY!

FatLossScience.org

24301027R00083

Made in the USA
Lexington, KY
15 July 2013